The Only *EKG Book* You'll Ever Need

The Only *EKG Book* You'll Ever Need

Second Edition

Malcolm S. Thaler, M.D.

Attending Physician
The Bryn Mawr Hospital
Bryn Mawr, Pennsylvania

J. B. Lippincott Company
Philadelphia

Acquisitions Editor: Richard Winters
Developmental Editor: Melissa James
Project Editor: Molly E. Dickmeyer
Indexer: Ann Cassar
Art Director: Susan Hermansen
Interior Deisgner: Anne O'Donnell
Cover Designer: Larry Pezzato
Production Manager: Caren Erlichman
Senior Production Coordinator: Kevin P. Johnson
Compositor: Tapsco, Incorporated
Printer/Binder: R. R. Donnelly/Crawfordsville
2nd Edition

Library of Congress Cataloging-in-Publication Data

Thaler, Malcolm S.
    The only EKG book you'll ever need/Malcolm S. Thaler.—2nd ed.
      p. cm.
    Inculdes index.
    ISBN 0-397-51408-5
    1. Electrocardiography. I. Title.
    [DNLM: 1. Electrocardiography. WG 140 T365o 1995
  RC638.5.E5T48 1995
  616.1'207547—dc20
  DNLM/DLC
  for Library of Congress

                94-33314
                CIP

6   5   4   3   2   1

Library of Congress Cataloging-in-Publications Data

⊚ This paper meets the requirements of ANSI/NISO Z39.48-1992 (permanence of paper).

The authors and publisher have exerted every effort to ensure that drug selection and dosage set forth in this text are in accord with current recommendations and practice at the time of publication. However, in view of ongoing research, changes in government regulations, and the constant flow of information relating to drug therapy and drug reactions, the reader is urged to check the package insert for each drug for any change in indications and dosage and for added warnings and precautions. This is particularly important when the recommended agent is a new or infrequently employed drug.

For **Nancy, Ali, and Jon,** altogether the heart of my matter

Preface

The warm and enthusiastic response of reviewers, teachers, and the many thousands of readers of the first edition of this textbook has been heard and gratefully received. When we first conceived this book, there was one overriding concern that guided the project: to teach the student to read an EKG quickly and accurately, and to do so simply, clearly, concisely, and with a sizable dollop of wit and good fun. As Gilbert and Sullivan's fool, Jack Point, correctly pointed out, "He who'd make his fellow creatures wise, should always gild the philosophic pill." Here, then, is the pill, primed, lacquered, and gilt, ready for easy digestion.

Preface to the First Edition

This book is about learning. It's about keeping simple things simple and complicated things clear, concise, and—yes, simple, too. It's about getting from here to there without scaring you to death, boring you to tears, or intimidating your socks off. It's about turning ignorance into knowledge, knowledge into wisdom, and all with a bit of fun.

Ultimately, of course, this book is about electrocardiography, still (if not more than ever) one of the most powerful clinical tools we have. Even if you have never seen an EKG before, you should emerge from this book a competent electrocardiographer, ready to tackle basic rhythm disturbances, diagnose heart attacks, and recognize a whole host of acute and chronic problems affecting the heart. **You will know what you need to know.**

There are, of course, many EKG texts currently available, most of them excellent, all with something important to offer. What we have tried to accomplish in *The Only EKG Book You'll Ever Need* is to provide in one place precisely the information you will need—no more and no less—to read EKGs rapidly and accurately. And just as importantly, each concept, each EKG, is discussed within its proper clinical context—the patient who is being studied. Along the way, many personal choices have had to be made about what to include and what to leave out, how deeply to explore a topic, and how best to express an idea; I hope that most of the choices have been good ones.

Acknowledgments

The remarkable efforts of several individuals deserve special mention. Glenn Haper, M.D., a superlative cardiologist and geniune mensch, helped bring this book into the new millenium with his tactful criticisms and prescient insights. Anyone who can draw a straight line immediately earns my admiration, and J. Brett McNaughton drew lots of straight lines (and some impressive curves, too) and drew them very well; his illustrations remained faithful to the first edition while adding a scholastic ornamental glamour of their own, and are a joy to behold. Also, very special thanks must be extended to all of the folks at J. B. Lippincott who put up with me for a second go-around. In particular, let me say a loud thank you to Richard Winters; we have seen many projects through together, and fortunately, we both have day jobs.

Contents

The Only *EKG Book* You'll Ever Need

The Only EKG Book You'll Ever Need, second edition, by Malcolm S. Thaler.
JB Lippincott Company, Philadelphia © 1995.

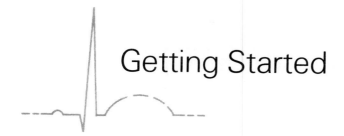

Getting Started

In this chapter you will learn:

1 not a thing, but don't worry. There is plenty to come. Here is your
chance to turn a few pages and get yourself settled and ready to roll.
Relax. Pour some tea. Begin.

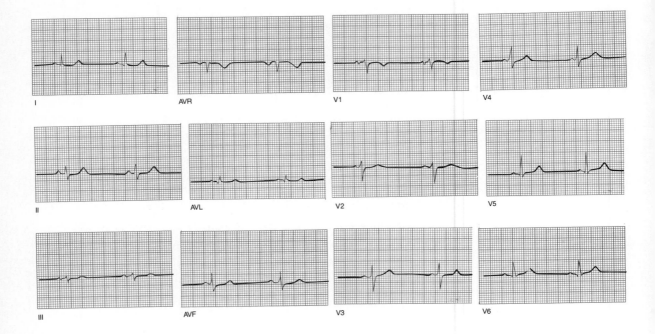

I
AVR
V1
V4

II
AVL
V2
V5

III
AVF
V3
V6

On the opposite page is a normal electrocardiogram, or EKG. By the time you have finished this book—and it won't take very much time at all—you will be able to recognize a normal EKG almost instantly. Perhaps even more importantly, you will have learned to spot all of the common abnormalities that can occur on an EKG, **and you will be good at it!**

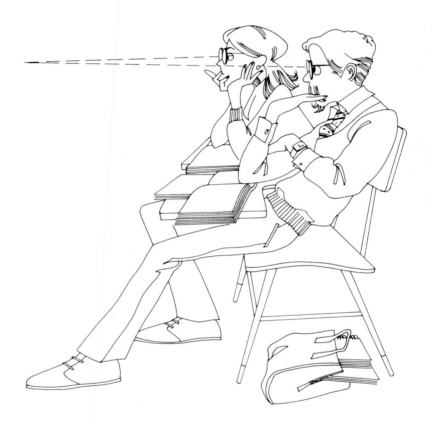

Some people have compared learning to read EKGs with learning to read music. In both instances, one is faced with a completely new notational system not rooted in conventional language and full of unfamiliar shapes and symbols.

But there really is no comparison. The simple lub-dub of the heart offers little challenge to the complexity of a Beethoven string quartet, a Mahler symphony, or even a Springsteen ballad.

There's just not that much going on.

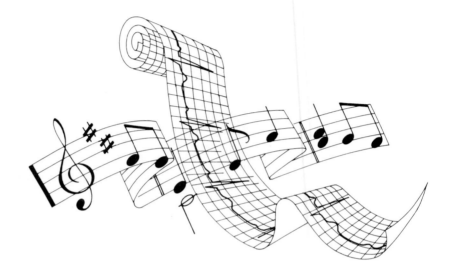

The EKG is a tool of remarkable clinical power, remarkable both for the ease with which it can be mastered and for the extraordinary range of situations in which it can provide helpful and, frequently, even critical information. One glance at an EKG can diagnose an evolving myocardial infarction, identify a potentially life-threatening arrhythmia, pinpoint the chronic effects of sustained hypertension or the acute effects of a massive pulmonary embolus, or simply provide a measure of reassurance to someone who wants to begin an exercise program.

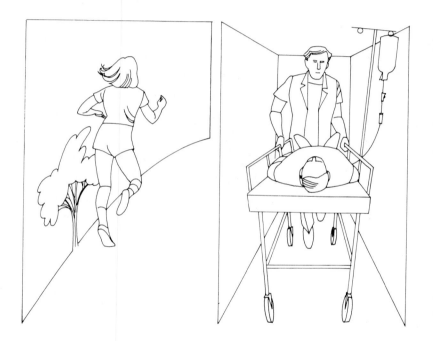

Remember, however, that the EKG is only a tool, and like any tool is only as capable as its user. Put a chisel in my hand and you are unlikely to get Michelangelo's David.

The eight chapters of this book will take you on an *electrifying* voyage from ignorance to dazzling competence. You will amaze your friends (and, more importantly, yourself). The roadmap you will follow looks like this:

Chapter 1: You will learn about the electrical events that generate the different waves on the EKG, and—armed with this knowledge—you will be able to recognize and understand the normal 12-lead EKG.

Chapter 2: You will see how simple and predictable alterations in certain waves permit the diagnosis of enlargement and hypertrophy of the atria and ventricles.

Chapter 3: You will become familiar with the most common disturbances in cardiac rhythm, and learn why some are life-threatening while others are merely nuisances.

Chapter 4: You will learn to identify interruptions in the normal pathways of cardiac conduction, and will be introduced to pacemakers.

Chapter 5: As a complement to chapter 4, you will learn what happens when the electrical current by-passes the usual channels of conduction and arrives more quickly at its destination.

Chapter 6: You will learn to diagnose a myocardial infarction (heart attack) and distinguish it from reversible angina.

Chapter 7: You will see how various *noncardiac* phenomena can alter the EKG.

Chapter 8: You will put all your new-found knowledge together into a simple 11-step method for reading all EKGs.

The whole process is straightforward and rather unsophisticated and should not be the least bit intimidating. Intricacies of thought and great leaps of creative logic are not required.

This is not the time for deep thinking.

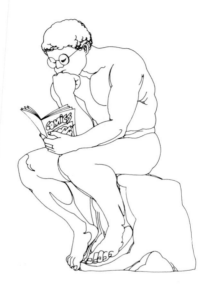

The Only EKG Book You'll Ever Need, second edition, by Malcolm S. Thaler.
JB Lippincott Company, Philadelphia © 1995.

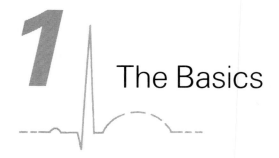

The Basics

In this chapter you will learn:

1 how the electrical current in the heart is generated

2 how this current is propagated through the four chambers of the heart

3 that the movement of electricity through the heart produces predictable wave patterns on the EKG

4 how the EKG machine detects and records these waves

5 that the EKG looks at the heart from 12 different perspectives

6 that you are now able to recognize and *understand* all the lines and waves on the 12-lead EKG.

⊞ *Electricity and the Heart*

Electricity, an innate biological electricity, is what makes the heart go. The EKG is nothing more than a recording of the heart's electrical activity, and it is through perturbations in the normal electrical patterns that we are able to diagnose many different cardiac disorders.

All You Need to Know About Cellular Electrophysiology in Two Pages

Cardiac cells, in their resting state, are electrically polarized, *i.e.,* their insides are negatively charged with respect to their outsides. This electrical polarity is maintained by membrane pumps that ensure the appropriate distribution of ions (primarily potassium, sodium, chloride, and calcium) necessary to keep the insides of these cells relatively electronegative.

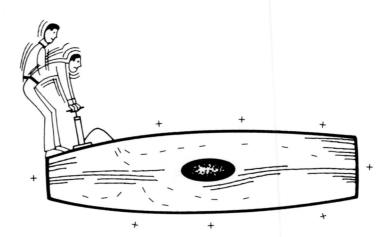

The resting cardiac cell maintains its electrical polarity by means of a membrane pump. This pump requires a constant supply of energy, and the gentleman above, were he real rather than a metaphor, would soon be flat on his back.

Cardiac cells can lose their internal negativity in a process called *depolarization*. **Depolarization is the fundamental electrical event of the heart.**

Depolarization is propagated from cell to cell, producing a wave of depolarization that can be transmitted across the entire heart. This wave of depolarization represents a flow of electricity, an electrical current, and can be detected by electrodes placed on the surface of the body.

After depolarization is complete, the cardiac cells are able to restore their resting polarity through a process called *repolarization*. This, too, can be sensed by recording electrodes.

All of the different waves that we see on an EKG are manifestations of these two processes: depolarization and repolarization.

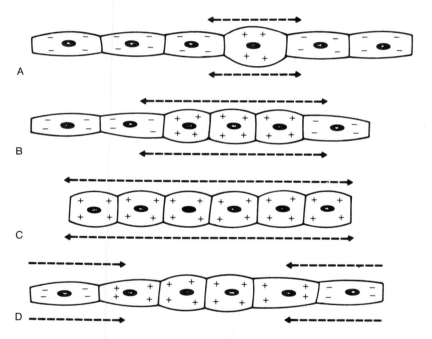

In *A,* a single cell has depolarized. A wave of depolarization then propagates from cell to cell (*B*) until all are depolarized (*C*). Repolarization (*D*) then restores each cell's normal polarity.

From the standpoint of the electrocardiographer, the heart consists of three types of cells:

- *Pacemaker cells*—the electrical power source of the heart

- *Electrical conducting cells*—the hard wiring of the heart

- *Myocardial cells*—the contractile machinery of the heart.

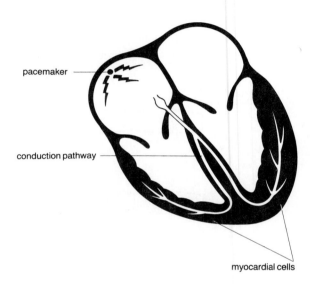

Pacemaker Cells

Pacemaker cells are small cells approximately 5 to 10 μm long. These cells are able to depolarize spontaneously over and over again, at a particular rate. The rate of depolarization is determined by the innate electrical characteristics of the cell and by external neural and hormonal input. Each spontaneous depolarization serves as the source of a wave of depolarization that initiates one complete cycle of cardiac contraction and relaxation.

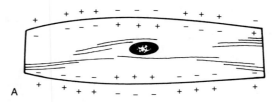

(*A*) A pacemaker cell depolarizing spontaneously.

If we record one electrical cycle of depolarization and repolarization from a single cell, we get an electrical tracing like that in **B.** This tracing is called an **action potential.**

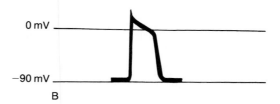

(*B*) The resultant action potential. With each spontaneous depolarization, a new action potential is generated, which in turn stimulates neighboring cells to depolarize, and so on, until the entire heart has been depolarized.

The dominant pacemaker cells in the heart are located high up in the right atrium. This group of cells is called the **sinoatrial (SA) node,** or **sinus node** for short. These cells typically fire at a rate of 60 to 100 times per minute, but the rate can vary tremendously depending upon the activity of the autonomic nervous system (sympathetic stimulation from adrenalin accelerates the sinus node, whereas vagal stimulation slows it) and the demands of the body for increased cardiac output (exercise raises the heart rate, whereas a restful afternoon nap lowers it).

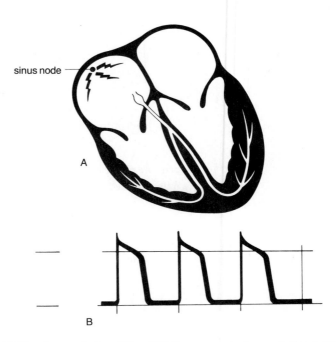

(*A*) The sinus node fires 60 to 100 times per minute, producing a regular series of action potentials (*B*), each of which initiates a wave of depolarization that will spread through the heart.

Electrical Conducting Cells

Electrical conducting cells are long, thin cells. Like the wires of an electrical circuit, these cells carry current rapidly and efficiently to distant regions of the heart. The ventricles are wired quite elaborately with these cells, but the existence of discrete conducting pathways in the atria is still disputed.

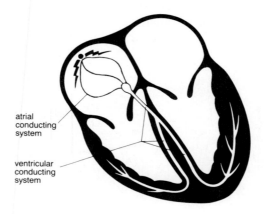

atrial
conducting
system

ventricular
conducting
system

The hard wiring of the heart. The ventricular conducting system has been precisely defined, but the existence of discrete atrial conducting pathways is still debated.

Myocardial Cells

The *myocardial cells* constitute by far the major part of the heart tissue. They are responsible for the heavy labor of repeatedly contracting and relaxing, thereby delivering blood to the rest of the body. These cells are about 50 to 100 μm in length and contain an abundance of the contractile proteins, actin and myosin.

When a wave of depolarization reaches a myocardial cell, calcium is released within the cell, causing the cell to contract. This process, in which calcium plays the key intermediary role, is called *excitation–contraction coupling*.

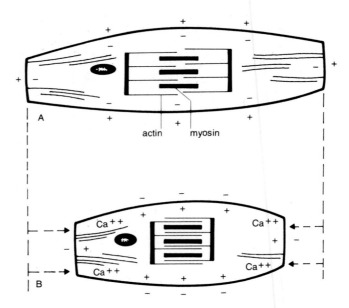

Depolarization causes calcium to be released within a myocardial cell. This influx of calcium allows actin and myosin, the contractile proteins, to interact, causing the cell to contract. (*A*) A resting myocardial cell. (*B*) A depolarized, contracted myocardial cell.

Myocardial cells can transmit an electrical current just like electrical conducting cells, but myocardial cells do so far less efficiently. Thus, a wave of depolarization, upon reaching the myocardial cells, will spread out slowly across the entire myocardium.

⊞ *Time and Voltage*

The waves that appear on an EKG primarily reflect the electrical activity of the *myocardial cells,* which comprise the vast bulk of the heart. Pacemaker activity and transmission by the conducting system are generally *not* seen on the EKG; these events simply do not generate sufficient voltage to be recorded by surface electrodes.

The waves produced by myocardial depolarization and repolarization are recorded on EKG paper and, like any type of wave, have three chief characteristics:

1. *Duration,* measured in fractions of a second

2. *Amplitude,* measured in millivolts (mV)

3. *Configuration,* a more subjective criterion referring to the shape and appearance of a wave.

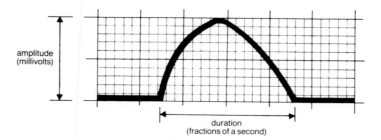

A typical wave that might be seen on any EKG. It is two large squares (or 10 small squares) in amplitude, three large squares (or 15 small squares) in duration, and slightly asymmetric in configuration.

EKG Paper

EKG paper is a long, continuous roll of graph paper, usually pink, with light and dark lines running vertically and horizontally. The light lines circumscribe small squares of 1 mm × 1 mm; the dark lines delineate large squares of 5 mm × 5 mm.

The horizontal axis measures time. The distance across one small square represents 0.04 seconds. The distance across one large square is five times greater, or 0.2 seconds.

The vertical axis measures voltage. The distance along one small square represents 0.1 mV, and along one large square, 0.5 mV.

You will need to memorize these numbers at some point, so you might as well do it now.

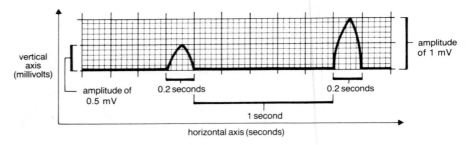

Both waves are one large square in duration (0.2 seconds), but the second wave is twice the voltage of the first (1 mV compared with 0.5 mV). The flat segment connecting the two waves is five large squares (5 × 0.2 seconds = 1 second) in duration.

P Waves, QRS Complexes, T Waves, and Some Straight Lines

Let's follow one cycle of cardiac contraction (systole) and relaxation (diastole), focusing on the electrical events that produce the basic waves and lines of the standard EKG.

Atrial Depolarization

The sinus node fires spontaneously (an event not visible on the EKG), and a wave of depolarization begins to spread outward into the atrial myocardium, much as if a pebble were dropped into a calm lake. Depolarization of the atrial myocardial cells results in atrial contraction.

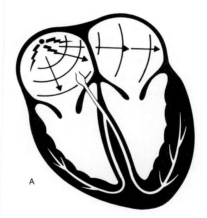

Each cycle of cardiac contraction and relaxation begins when the sinus node depolarizes spontaneously. (*A*) The wave of depolarization then propagates through both atria, causing them to contract.

During atrial depolarization and contraction, electrodes placed on the surface of the body will record a small burst of electrical activity lasting a fraction of a second. This is the *P wave*. It is a recording of the spread of depolarization through the atrial myocardium from start to finish.

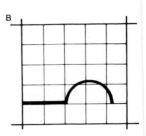

(*B*) The EKG records a small deflection.

Because the sinus node is located in the right atrium, the right atrium begins to depolarize before the left atrium and finishes earlier as well. Therefore, the first part of the P wave predominantly represents right atrial depolarization, and the second part left atrial depolarization.

Once atrial depolarization is complete, the EKG again becomes electrically silent.

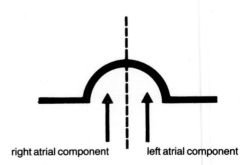

right atrial component   left atrial component

The P Wave

A Pause Separates the Atria From the Ventricles

In healthy hearts, there is an electrical gate at the junction of the atria and the ventricles. The wave of depolarization, having completed its journey through the atria, now encounters a barrier. Here, a structure called the *atrioventricular (AV) node* slows conduction to a crawl. This pause lasts only a fraction of a second.

This physiologic delay in conduction is essential to allow the atria to finish contracting before the ventricles begin to contract. This clever electrical wiring of the heart permits the atria to empty their volume of blood completely into the ventricles before the ventricles contract.

Like the sinus node, the AV node is also under the influence of the autonomic nervous system. Vagal stimulation slows the current even further, whereas sympathetic stimulation accelerates the current.

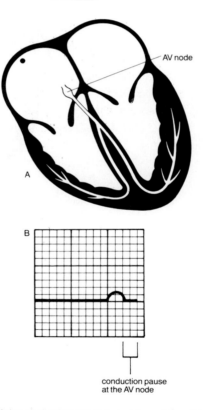

(*A*) The wave of depolarization is briefly held up at the AV node. (*B*) During this pause, the EKG falls silent; there is no detectable electrical activity.

Ventricular Depolarization

After about one tenth of a second, the depolarizing wave escapes the AV node and is swept rapidly down the ventricles along specialized electrical conducting cells.

This ventricular conducting system has a complex anatomy, but essentially consists of three parts:

1. Bundle of His

2. Bundle branches

3. Terminal Purkinje fibers.

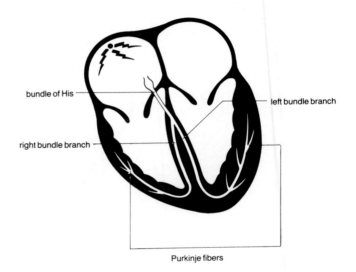

bundle of His

left bundle branch

right bundle branch

Purkinje fibers

The *bundle of His* emerges from the AV node and almost immediately divides into right and left bundle branches. The *right bundle branch* carries the current down the right side of the interventricular septum all the way to the apex of the right ventricle. The *left bundle branch* is more complicated. It divides into three major fascicles:

1. *Septal fascicle*, which depolarizes the interventricular septum (the wall of muscle separating the right and left ventricles) in a left-to-right direction.

2. *Anterior fascicle*, which runs along the anterior surface of the left ventricle.

3. *Posterior fascicle*, which sweeps over the posterior surface of the left ventricle.

The right bundle branch and the left bundle branch and its fascicles terminate in countless tiny *Purkinje fibers*, which resemble tiny twigs coming off the branches of a tree. These fibers deliver the electrical current into the ventricular myocardium.

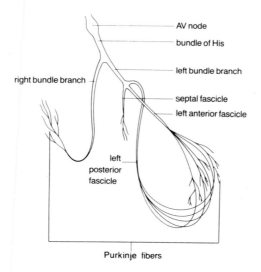

The ventricular conduction system, shown in detail. Below the bundle of His, the conduction system divides into right and left bundle branches. The right bundle branch remains intact, whereas the left divides into three separate fascicles.

The beginning of ventricular myocardial depolarization—and, hence, ventricular contraction—is marked by a new deflection on the EKG called the *QRS complex*. The amplitude of the QRS complex is much greater than that of the atrial P wave, because the ventricles are so much larger than the atria. The QRS complex is also more complicated and variable in shape, reflecting the greater intricacy of the pathway of ventricular depolarization.

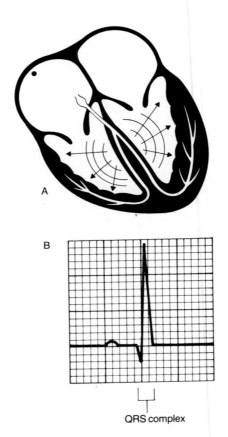

QRS complex

(*A*) Ventricular depolarization generates (*B*) a complicated waveform on the EKG called the QRS complex.

The Parts of the QRS Complex

The QRS complex consists of several distinct waves, each of which has a name. Because the precise configuration of the QRS complex can vary so greatly, a standard format for naming each component has been devised. It may seem a bit arbitrary to you right now, but it actually makes good sense.

1. If the first deflection is downward, it is called a *Q wave*.

2. The first upward deflection is called an *R wave*.

3. If there is a second upward deflection, it is called *R′* (R-prime).

4. The first downward deflection following an upward deflection is called an *S wave*. Therefore, if the first wave of the complex is an R wave then the ensuing downward deflection is called an S wave, not a Q wave. A downward deflection can only be called a Q wave if it is the first wave of the complex. Any other downward deflection is called an S wave.

   Here are several of the most common QRS configurations, with each wave component named.

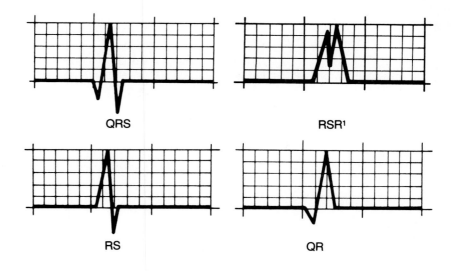

QRS

RSR¹

RS

QR

The earliest part of the QRS complex represents depolarization of the interventricular septum by the septal fascicle of the left bundle branch. The right and left ventricles then depolarize at about the same time, but most of what we see on the EKG represents left ventricular activation, because the muscle mass of the left ventricle is about three times that of the right ventricle.

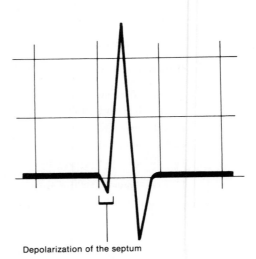

Depolarization of the septum

The initial part of the QRS complex represents septal depolarization. Sometimes, this septal depolarization may appear as a small, discrete, negative deflection, a Q wave.

Repolarization

After myocardial cells depolarize, they pass through a brief refractory period during which they are resistant to further stimulation. They then *repolarize,* that is, they restore the electronegativity of their interiors so that they can be restimulated.

Just as there is a wave of depolarization, there is also a wave of repolarization. This, too, can be seen on the EKG. Ventricular repolarization inscribes a third wave on the EKG, the *T wave.*

Note: There is a wave of atrial repolarization as well, but it coincides with ventricular depolarization and is hidden by the much more prominent QRS complex.

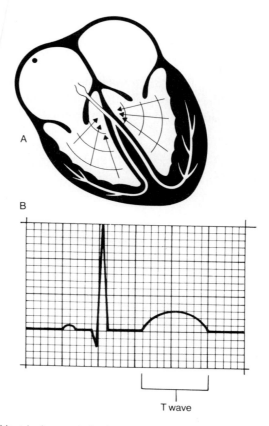

(*A*) Ventricular repolarization generates (*B*) T wave on the EKG.

⊞ *Naming the Straight Lines*

The different straight lines connecting the various waves have also been given names. Thus, we speak of the *PR interval,* the *ST segment,* and the *QT interval.*

What differentiates a segment from an interval? A segment is a straight line connecting two waves, whereas an interval encompasses at least one wave plus the connecting straight line.

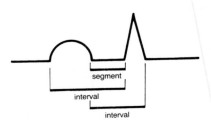

The *PR interval* includes the P wave and the straight line connecting it to the QRS complex. It therefore measures the time from the start of atrial depolarization to the start of ventricular depolarization.

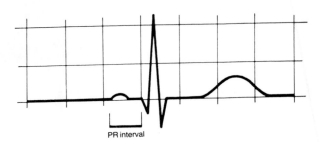

The *ST segment* is the straight line connecting the end of the QRS complex with the beginning of the T wave. It measures the time from the end of ventricular depolarization to the start of ventricular repolarization.

The *QT interval* includes the QRS complex, the ST segment, and the T wave. It therefore measures the time from the beginning of ventricular depolarization to the end of ventricular repolarization.

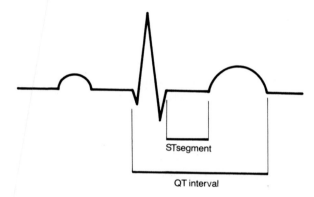

STsegment

QT interval

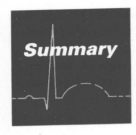

The Waves and Straight Lines of the EKG

1. Each cycle of cardiac contraction and relaxation is initiated by spontaneous depolarization of the sinus node. This event is not seen on the EKG.

2. The P wave records atrial depolarization and contraction. The first part of the P wave reflects right atrial activity; the second part reflects left atrial activity.

3. There is a brief pause when the electrical current reaches the AV node, and the EKG falls silent.

4. The wave of depolarization then spreads along the ventricular conducting system (His bundle, bundle branches, and Purkinje fibers) and out into the ventricular myocardium. The first part of the ventricles to be depolarized is the interventricular septum. Ventricular depolarization generates the QRS complex.

5. The T wave records ventricular repolarization. Atrial repolarization is not seen.

6. Various segments and intervals describe the time between these events:

   a. The PR interval measures the time from the start of atrial depolarization to the start of ventricular depolarization.

   b. The ST segment records the time from the end of ventricular depolarization to the start of ventricular repolarization.

   c. The QT interval measures the time from the start of ventricular depolarization to the end of ventricular repolarization.

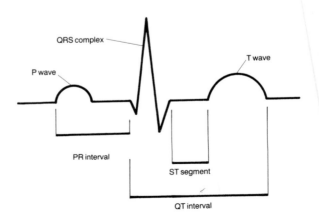

⊞ *Making Waves*

Electrodes can be placed anywhere on the surface of the body in order to record the heart's electrical activity. If we do this, we quickly discover that the waves recorded by a positive electrode on the left arm look very different from those recorded by a positive electrode on the right arm (or right leg, left leg, etc.).

It's easy to see why this occurs. A wave of depolarization moving *toward* a positive electrode causes a *positive* deflection on the EKG. A wave of depolarization moving *away* from a positive electrode causes a *negative* deflection.

Look at the figure below. The wave of depolarization is moving left to right, *toward* the electrode. The EKG records a positive deflection.

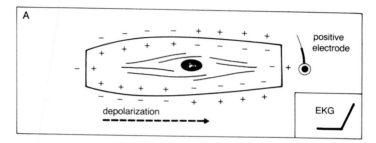

(*A*) A wave of depolarization moving toward a positive electrode records a positive deflection on the EKG.

Now look at the following figure. The wave of depolarization is moving right to left; the electrode is now placed so that the wave of depolarization is moving *away* from it. The EKG therefore records a negative deflection.

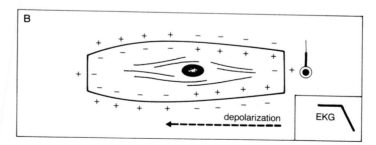

(*B*) A wave of depolarization moving away from a positive electrode records a negative deflection on the EKG.

What will the EKG record if the positive electrode is placed in the middle of the cell?

Initially, as the wavefront approaches the electrode, the EKG records a positive deflection.

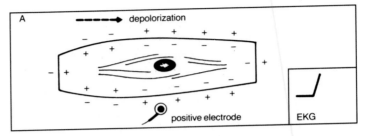

Depolarization moving perpendicularly to a positive electrode generates a biphasic wave on the EKG. (*A*) Depolarization begins, generating a positive deflection on the EKG.

Then, at the precise moment that the wave reaches the electrode, the positive and negative charges are balanced and essentially cancel each other out. The EKG recording returns to baseline.

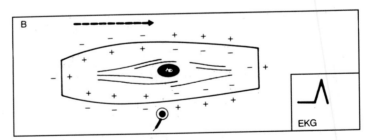

(*B*) The wavefront reaches the electrode. The positive and negative charges are balanced, and the EKG returns to baseline.

As the wave of depolarization recedes, a negative deflection is inscribed.

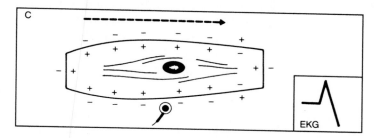

(*C*) The wave of depolarization begins to recede from the electrode, generating a negative deflection.

The EKG finally returns to baseline once again when the entire muscle is depolarized.

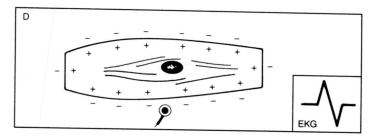

(*D*) The cell is fully depolarized, and the EKG once again returns to baseline.

The final inscription of a depolarizing wave moving perpendicularly to a positive electrode is a *biphasic wave.*

The effects of repolarization on the EKG are similar to those of depolarization, except that the charges are reversed. A wave of repolarization moving *toward* a positive electrode inscribes a *negative* deflection on the EKG. A wave of repolarization moving away from a positive electrode produces a *positive* deflection on the EKG. A perpendicular wave produces a *biphasic wave;* however, the negative deflection of the biphasic wave now *precedes* the positive deflection.

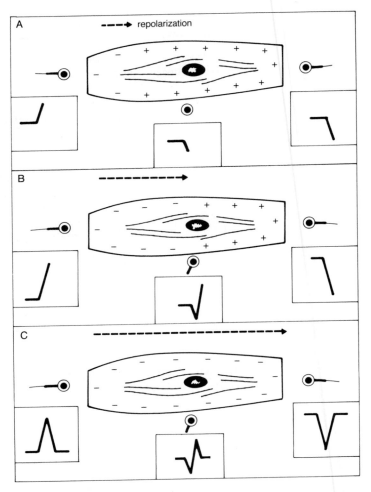

A wave of repolarization moving through muscle tissue is recorded by three different positive electrodes. (*A*) Early repolarization. (*B*) Late repolarization. (*C*) Repolarization is complete.

We can easily apply these concepts to the entire heart. Electrodes placed on the surface of the body will record waves of depolarization and repolarization as they sweep through the heart.

If a wave of depolarization passing through the heart is moving toward a surface electrode, that electrode will record a positive deflection (electrode *A*). If the wave of depolarization is moving away from the electrode, the electrode will record a negative deflection (electrode *B*). If the wave of depolarization is moving perpendicularly to the electrode, the electrode will record a biphasic wave (electrode *C*). The effects of repolarization are precisely the opposite of those of depolarization, as you would expect.

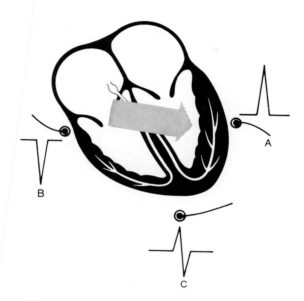

A wave of depolarization moving through the heart *(large arrow)*. Electrode *A* records a positive deflection, electrode *B* records a negative deflection, and electrode *C* records a biphasic wave.

⊞ The 12 Views of the Heart

If the heart was as simple as a single myocardial cell, a couple of recording electrodes would give us all the information we need to describe its electrical activity. However, as we have already seen, the heart is *not* so simple—a burden to you, a boon to authors of EKG books.

The heart is a three-dimensional organ, and its electrical activity must be understood in three dimensions as well. A couple of electrodes are not adequate to do this, a fact that the original electrocardiographers recognized nearly a century ago when they devised the first limb leads. Today, the standard EKG consists of 12 leads, with each lead determined by the placement and orientation of various electrodes on the body. Each lead views the heart at a unique angle, enhancing its sensitivity to a particular region of the heart at the expense of others. The more views, the more information is provided.

To read an EKG and extract as much information as possible, you need to understand the 12-lead system.

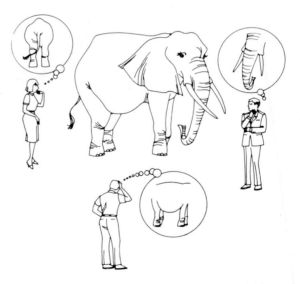

Three observers get three very different impressions of this consummate example of the *Loxodonta africana*. One observer sees the trunk, another sees the body, and the third sees the tail. If you wanted the best description of the elephant, who would you ask? All three, of course.

To prepare a patient for a 12-lead EKG, two electrodes are placed on the wrists and two on the ankles. These provide the basis for the six *limb leads,* which include the three *standard leads* and the three *augmented leads* (these terms will make more sense in a moment). Six electrodes are also placed across the chest, forming the six *precordial leads.*

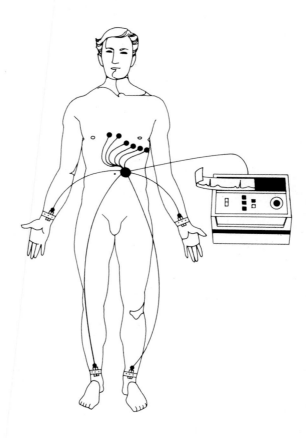

The Six Limb Leads

The limb leads view the heart in a vertical plane called the *frontal plane*. The frontal plane can be envisioned as a giant circle superimposed on the patient's body. This circle is then marked off in degrees. The limb leads view electrical forces (waves of depolarization and repolarization) moving up and down and left and right through this circle.

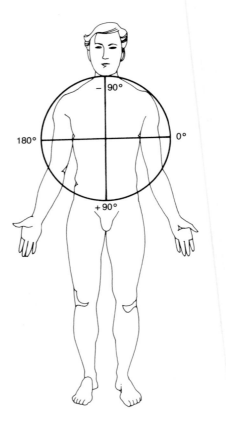

The frontal plane is a coronal plane. The limb leads view electrical forces moving up and down and left and right on the frontal plane.

To produce the six leads of the frontal plane, each of the electrodes is variably designated as positive or negative (this is actually done automatically by circuitry inside the EKG machine).

Each lead has its own specific view of the heart, or *angle of orientation*. The angle of each lead can be determined by drawing a line from the negative electrode to the positive electrode. The resultant angle is then expressed in degrees by superimposing it on the 360° circle of the frontal plane.

The three standard limb leads are defined as follows:

1. Lead I is created by making the left arm positive and the right arm negative. Its angle of orientation is 0°.

2. Lead II is created by making the legs positive and the right arm negative. Its angle of orientation is 60°.

3. Lead III is created by making the legs positive and the left arm negative. Its angle of orientation is 120°.

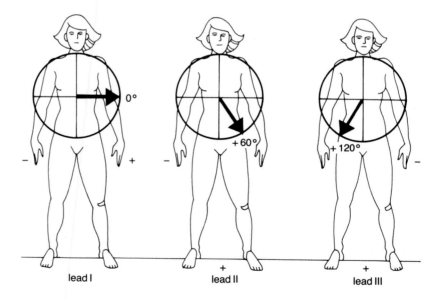

The three augmented limb leads are created somewhat differently. A single lead is chosen to be positive and all the others are made negative, with their average essentially serving as the negative electrode (common ground). They are called *augmented leads* because the EKG machinery must amplify the tracings to get an adequate recording.

1. Lead AVL is created by making the left arm positive and the other limbs negative. Its angle of orientation is −30°.

2. Lead AVR is created by making the right arm positive and the other limbs negative. Its angle of orientation is −150°.

3. Lead AVF is created by making the legs positive and the other limbs negative. Its angle of orientation is +90°.

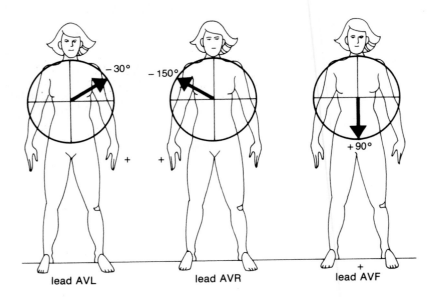

lead AVL   lead AVR   lead AVF

In the figure below, all six leads of the frontal plane are indicated with their appropriate angles of orientation. Just as our three observers each looked at the elephant from his or her own unique perspective, so each lead perceives the heart from its own unique point of view.

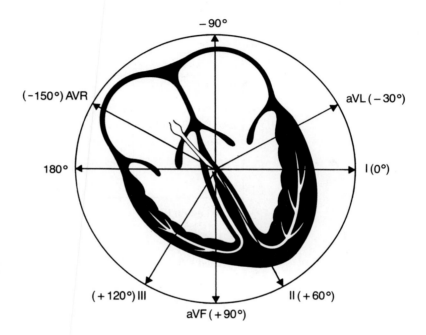

Leads II, III, and AVF are called the *inferior leads* because they most effectively view the inferior surface of the heart.

Leads I and AVL are often called the *left lateral leads* because they have the best view of the left lateral wall of the heart.

AVR is pretty much a loner, and you can call it whatever you like.

Memorize these six leads and their angles.

Lead	Angle	
Inferior Leads		
Lead II	+60°	
Lead III	+120°	
Lead AVF	+90°	
Left Lateral Leads		
Lead I	+0°	
Lead AVL	-30°	
Lead AVR	-150°	

Of six limb leads, three are standard (I, II, and III), and three are augmented (AVR, AVL, and AVF). Each lead views the heart from its own particular angle of orientation.

The Six Precordial Leads

The six precordial leads, or chest leads, are even easier to understand. They are arranged across the chest in a *horizontal plane* as illustrated below. Whereas the leads of the frontal plane view electrical forces moving up and down and left and right, the precordial leads record forces moving anteriorly and posteriorly.

To create the six precordial leads, each chest electrode is made positive in turn, and the whole body is taken as the common ground. The six positive electrodes, creating the precordial leads V_1 through V_6, are positioned as follows:

- V_1 is placed in the fourth intercostal space to the right of the sternum.

- V_2 is placed in the fourth intercostal space to the left of the sternum.

- V_3 is placed between V_2 and V_4.

- V_4 is placed in the fifth intercostal space in the midclavicular line.

- V_5 is placed between V_4 and V_6.

- V_6 is placed in the fifth intercostal space in the midaxillary line.

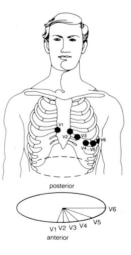

The precordial leads define a horizontal or transverse plane, and view electrical forces moving anteriorly and posteriorly.

Just like the limb leads, each precordial lead has its own particular line of sight and region of the heart that it views best.

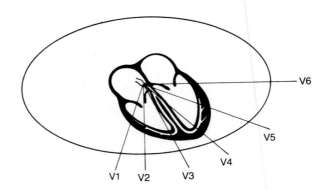

Note that the right ventricle lies anteriorly and medially, and the left ventricle lies posteriorly and laterally. Leads V_1 and V_2 lie directly over the right ventricle, V_3 and V_4 over the interventricular septum, and V_5 and V_6 over the left ventricle.

Leads V_1 through V_4 are often referred to as the *anterior leads*, and V_5 and V_6 join I and AVL as *left lateral leads*.

Leads	Group
V_1, V_2, V_3, V_4	Anterior
I, AVL, V_5, V_6	Left lateral
II, III, AVF	Inferior
AVR	—

A Word About Vectors

It is important to recognize that each EKG electrode records only the *average* current flow at any given moment. Thus, although tiny swirls of current may simultaneously be going off in every direction, each lead records only the instantaneous average of these forces. In this way, out of chaos, some very simple patterns emerge.

This concept is really quite simple; an analogy may help promote understanding. During the course of a soccer match, a goalie may kick or toss the ball many different times to various members of his team. Some balls will go to his or her left, others to his or her right, still others will go straight down the field. However, by the end of the game, the *average direction* of all of his or her kicks and tosses is likely to be straight ahead, toward the opposing net. This average movement can be represented by a single arrow, or *vector*.

This vector is precisely what our EKG electrodes record when measuring the electrical flow within the heart. The vector's angle of orientation represents the average *direction* of current flow, and its length represents the maximal voltage (*amplitude*) attained.

At any given moment, the electrical forces moving within the heart can be represented by a single vector, and this vector is translated by each of the 12 leads into the simple wave patterns that we see on the EKG.

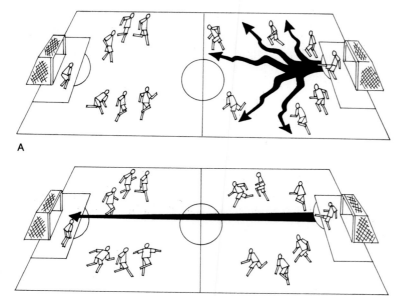

(*A*) The directions of each of the goalie's kicks during the course of the game. (*B*) A single vector represents the average direction of all of these kicks.

⊞ *The Normal 12-Lead EKG*

You now know the three things necessary to derive the normal 12-lead EKG:

1. The normal pathway of cardiac electrical activation and the names of the segments, waves, and intervals that are generated

2. The orientation of all 12 leads, six in the frontal plane and six in the horizontal plane

3. The simple concept that each lead records the average current flow at any given moment.

All we need to do now is to take what you already know and figure out what each wave looks like in each of the 12 leads.

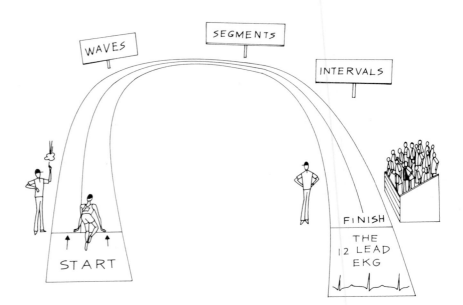

The P Wave

Atrial depolarization begins at the sinus node, high up in the right atrium. The right atrium depolarizes first, then the left atrium depolarizes. The average vector of current flow therefore points from right to left and slightly inferiorly (*large arrow*).

Any lead that views the wave of atrial depolarization as moving toward it will record a positive deflection on the EKG paper. The left lateral and inferior leads clearly fit this description. In the *frontal plane,* these leads include the left lateral leads I and AVL and the inferior leads II and AVF.

Lead III, which is also one of the inferior leads, is positioned a bit differently. It is the most rightward (orientation +120°) of the inferior leads and actually lies nearly perpendicular to the atrial current. Predictably, lead III frequently records a biphasic P wave.

Lead AVR, the most rightward of all the leads of the frontal plane (orientation −150°), sees the electrical current as moving away, so it records a purely negative deflection.

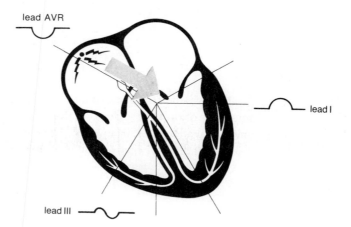

The vector of atrial depolarization points leftward and inferiorly. Therefore, lead I records a positive wave, AVR records a negative wave, and lead III records a biphasic wave.

In the *horizontal plane,* the left lateral leads V_5 and V_6 record a positive deflection, just as leads I and AVL did in the frontal plane. Lead V_1, lying over the right heart, is oriented perpendicularly to the direction of current flow and records a biphasic wave, just like lead III. Leads V_2 through V_4 are variable.

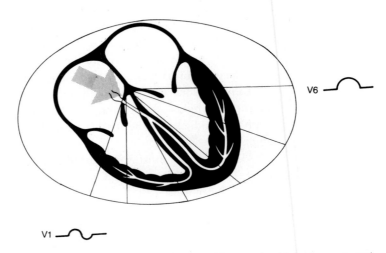

Atrial depolarization in a horizontal plane. V_1 records a biphasic wave, and V_6 records a positive wave.

Because the atria are small, the voltage they can generate is also small. The amplitude of the P wave does not normally exceed 0.25 mV (2.5 mm, or two and one half small squares) in any lead. The P wave amplitude is usually most positive in lead II and most negative in lead AVR.

But People Are Individuals

A word of caution is needed. Variations in anatomy and orientation of the heart from person to person make absolute rules impossible. For example, although the P wave in lead III is usually biphasic, it is not uncommon for it to be negative in perfectly normal hearts. All it takes is a change of a few degrees in the vector of current flow to turn a biphasic wave into a negative one. This can happen, for instance, if the patient's heart is angled slightly differently in the chest cavity.

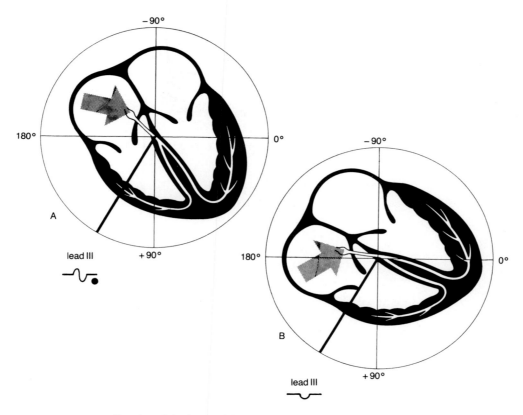

Rotation of the heart within the chest cavity redirects the perceived direction of current flow. Lead III is normally oriented perpendicularly to atrial depolarization. With the apex of the heart turned leftward, lead III will view atrial depolarization as receding and will record a wave that is largely negative.

The PR Interval

The PR interval represents the time from the start of atrial depolarization to the start of ventricular depolarization. It includes the delay in conduction that occurs at the AV node. The PR interval normally lasts from 0.12 to 0.2 seconds (3 mm to 5 mm on the EKG paper).

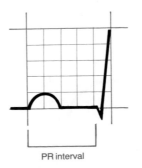

PR interval

The normal PR interval lasts from 0.12 to 0.2 seconds.

The QRS Complex Is Complex, but Not Complicated

Our wave of electrical depolarization, emerging from the AV node, is now ready to enter the ventricles.

Septal Q Waves

The interventricular septum, the wall of muscle separating the right and left ventricles, is the first to depolarize, and it does so in a left-to-right direction. The tiny septal fascicle of the left bundle branch is responsible for rapidly delivering the wave of depolarization to this region of the heart.

Septal depolarization is not always visible on the EKG, but when it is, this small left-to-right depolarization inscribes a tiny negative deflection in one or several of the left lateral leads. This initial negative deflection, or Q wave, may therefore be seen in leads I, AVL, V_5 and V_6. In some people, small Q waves can also be seen in the inferior leads.

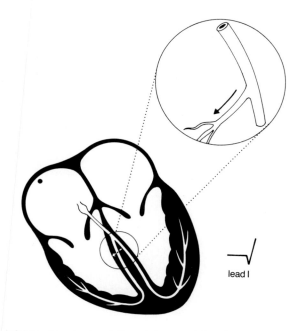

lead I

The left lateral leads view left-to-right septal depolarization as moving away; therefore, they record a small initial negative deflection, or Q wave. Small Q waves are also sometimes seen in the inferior leads; these are normal.

The Rest of the Ventricular Myocardium Depolarizes

The remainder of the ventricles, which comprises the vast bulk of the myocardium, depolarizes next. Because the left ventricle is so much larger than the right ventricle, it dominates the remainder of the QRS complex, and the average vector of current flow swings leftward. Normally, this vector points anywhere from 0° to +90°. In the frontal plane, therefore, large positive deflections (R waves) may be seen in many of the left lateral and inferior leads. Lead AVR, lying rightward, records a deep negative deflection (S wave).

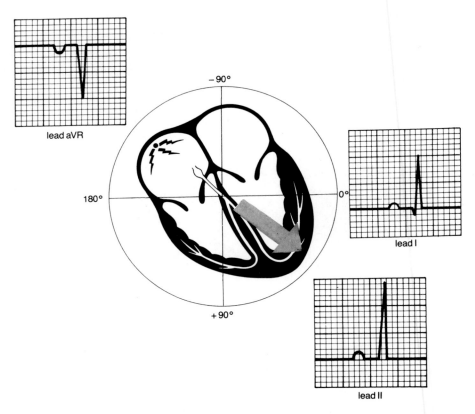

Ventricular depolarization as seen in leads I, II, and AVR. Lead I records a small Q wave due to septal depolarization and a tall R wave. Lead II also records a tall R wave and, less often, a small Q wave. The QRS complex in lead AVR is also deeply negative.

In the horizontal plane, leads V_1 and V_2, which overlie the right ventricle, record deep S waves, because the current is moving leftward, away from them. Conversely, leads V_5 and V_6, lying over the left ventricle, record tall positive R waves. Leads V_3 and V_4 represent a *transition zone,* and usually one of these leads records a biphasic wave, that is, an R wave and an S wave of nearly equal amplitude.

This pattern of progressively increasing R wave amplitude moving right to left in the precordial leads is called *R wave progression.* Lead V_1 has the smallest R wave; lead V_5, the largest (the R wave in lead V_6 is usually a little smaller than that in lead V_5). We also speak of a *transition zone,* the precordial lead or leads in which the QRS complex goes from being predominantly negative to predominantly positive. The normal transition zone occurs at leads V_3 and V_4.

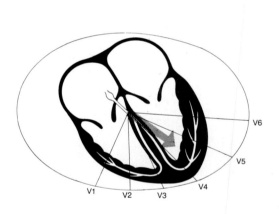
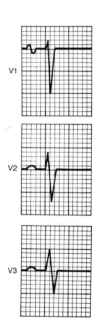
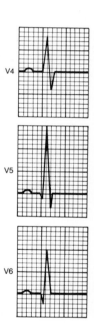

Ventricular depolarization in the precordial leads. Note the normal pattern of R wave progression. The wave in lead V_3 is biphasic.

A normal QRS complex is 0.06 to 0.1 seconds in duration. The amplitude of the QRS complex is much greater than that of the P wave, because the ventricles are so much larger and can support a much greater electrical potential.

The ST Segment

The ST segment is usually horizontal or gently upsloping in all leads. It represents the time from the end of ventricular depolarization to the start of ventricular repolarization.

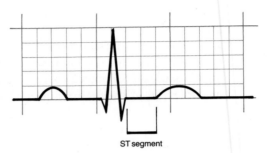

ST segment

The T Wave

The T wave represents ventricular *repolarization.*

Unlike depolarization, which is largely passive, repolarization requires the expenditure of a great deal of cellular energy (remember the membrane pump). The T wave is highly susceptible to all kinds of influences, both cardiac and noncardiac (*e.g.,* hormonal, neurologic), and is therefore variable in its appearance.

Nevertheless, certain general statements can be made. In the normal heart, repolarization usually begins in the last area of the heart to have been depolarized, and then travels backward, in a direction opposite that of the wave of depolarization (*large arrow*). Because both an approaching wave of depolarization and a receding wave of repolarization generate a positive deflection on the EKG, the same electrodes that recorded a *positive* deflection during *depolarization* (appearing as a tall R wave) will also generally record a *positive* deflection during *repolarization* (appearing as a positive T wave). **It is therefore typical and normal to find positive T waves in the same leads that have tall R waves.**

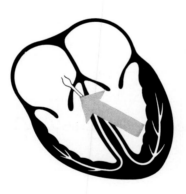
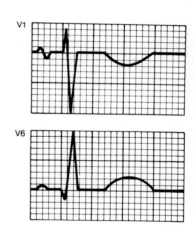

Ventricular repolarization generates the T wave on the EKG. The T wave is usually positive in leads with tall R waves.

The QT Interval

The QT interval encompasses the time from the beginning of ventricular depolarization to the end of ventricular repolarization. It therefore includes all of the electrical events that take place in the ventricles. From the standpoint of time, more of the QT interval is devoted to ventricular *repolarization* than depolarization (*i.e.*, the T wave is wider than the QRS complex).

The duration of the QT interval is proportionate to the heart rate. The faster the heart beats, the faster it must repolarize to prepare for the next contraction and, thus, the shorter the QT interval. Conversely, when the heart is beating slowly, there is little urgency to repolarize, and the QT interval is long. In general, the QT interval comprises approximately 40% of the normal cardiac cycle, as measured from one R wave to the next.

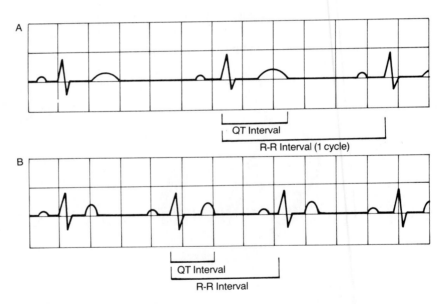

The QT interval comprises about 40% of each cardiac cycle (R-R interval). The faster the heart beats, the shorter the QT interval. The heart rate in *B* is considerably faster than that in *A*, and the QT interval is correspondingly much shorter (less than one and one half boxes versus two full boxes).

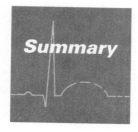

Summary

Orientation of the Waves of the Normal EKG

1. The P wave is small and usually positive in the left lateral and inferior leads. It is often biphasic in leads III and V_1. It is usually most positive in lead II and most negative in lead AVR.

2. The QRS complex is large, and tall R waves (positive deflections) are usually seen in most left lateral and inferior leads. R wave progression refers to the sequential enlargement of R waves as one proceeds across the precordial leads from V_1 to V_5. A small initial Q wave, representing septal depolarization, can often be seen in one or several of the left lateral leads, and sometimes in the inferior leads.

3. The T wave is variable, but it is usually positive in leads with tall R waves.

Now, take a good look at the following EKG. Does it seem familiar?

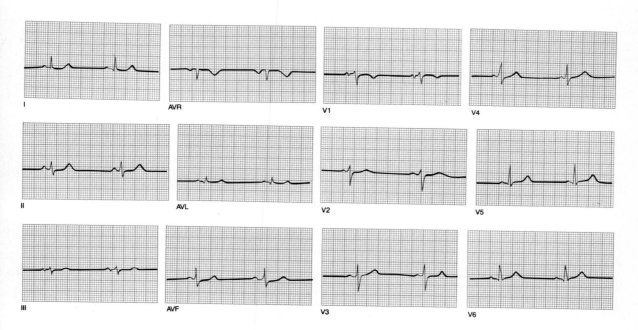

Of course it seems familiar. It's a normal 12-lead EKG, identical to the one that began the book.

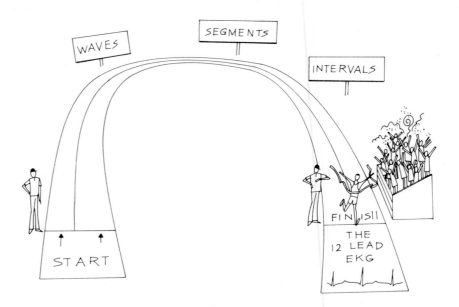

Congratulations! You have successfully traversed the most difficult terrain in this book. Everything that follows builds logically from the few basic principles you have now mastered.

⊞ *Coming Attractions*

You are now ready to use the EKG to diagnose an extraordinary variety of cardiac and noncardiac disorders. We shall group these disorders into five categories.

Hypertrophy and Enlargement (Chapter 2). The EKG can reveal whether a particular atrial or ventricular chamber is enlarged or hypertrophied. Valvular diseases or severe, sustained hypertension can affect the heart in this way, and the EKG can therefore help to recognize and evaluate these disorders.

Abnormalities of Rhythm (Chapter 3). The heart can beat too fast or too slow, fibrillate chaotically, or come to a sudden standstill. The EKG is still the best means to assess such rhythm disturbances, which, at their most severe, can lead to sudden death.

Abnormalities of Conduction (Chapters 4 and 5). If the normal pathways of cardiac electrical conduction become blocked, the heart rate can fall precipitously. The result can be *syncope,* a faint caused by a sudden decrease in cardiac output. Syncope is one of the leading causes of hospital admission. Conduction can also be accelerated along short circuits that bypass the normal delay in the AV node; we will look at these, too.

Myocardial Infarction (Chapter 6). The diagnosing of a myocardial infarction, or heart attack, is one of the most important roles for the EKG. There are many reasons why a patient may have chest pain, and the EKG can help sort these out.

Electrolyte Disturbances, Drug Effects, and Miscellaneous Disorders (Chapter 7). Various electrolyte disorders can affect cardiac conduction and even lead to sudden death if untreated. Medications such as digitalis, antidepressants, and antiarrhythmic agents can profoundly alter the EKG. A number of cardiac and noncardiac diseases can also cause dramatic shifts in the EKG. In each of these instances, a timely glance at an EKG may be diagnostic and sometimes lifesaving.

The Only EKG Book You'll Ever Need, second edition, by Malcolm S. Thaler.
JB Lippincott Company, Philadelphia © 1995.

2

Hypertrophy and Enlargement of the Heart

In this chapter you will learn:

1 what happens to a wave on the EKG when an atrium enlarges or a ventricle hypertrophies

2 the meaning of *electrical axis,* and its importance in diagnosing hypertrophy and enlargement

3 the criteria for the EKG diagnosis of right and left atrial enlargement

4 the criteria for the EKG diagnosis of right and left ventricular hypertrophy

5 the importance of recognizing a pattern of *strain* on the EKG of patients with severe ventricular hypertrophy

6 about the cases of Mildred W. and Tom L., which will test your ability to recognize the EKG changes of hypertrophy and enlargement.

⊞ *Definitions*

The term *hypertrophy* refers to an increase in muscle mass. The wall of a hypertrophied ventricle is thick and powerful. Hypertrophy is caused by *pressure overload*, in which the heart is forced to pump blood against an increased resistance, as in patients with systemic hypertension or aortic stenosis. Just as a weight lifter develops powerful pectoral muscles as he bench presses progressively heavier and heavier weights, so the heart muscle grows thicker and stronger as it is called on to eject blood against increasing resistance.

Enlargement refers to dilatation of a particular chamber. An enlarged ventricle can hold more blood than a normal ventricle. Enlargement is typically caused by *volume overload;* the chamber dilates to accommodate an increased amount of blood. Enlargement is most often seen with certain valvular diseases. Aortic insufficiency, for example, may cause left ventricular enlargement, and mitral insufficiency may result in left atrial enlargement.

Enlargement and hypertrophy frequently coexist. This is not surprising because both represent ways in which the heart tries to increase its cardiac output.

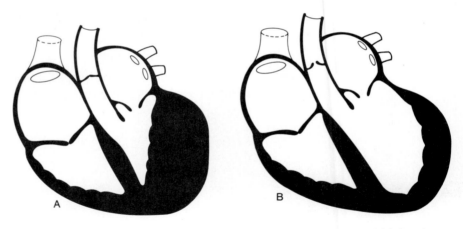

(*A*) A hypertrophied left ventricle caused by aortic stenosis. The wall is so thick that the chamber size is actually diminished. (*B*) An enlarged left ventricle. The chamber is bigger, but the wall thickness is normal.

The EKG is not very good at distinguishing between hypertrophy and enlargement. However, it is traditional to speak of *atrial enlargement* and *ventricular hypertrophy* when reading EKGs.*

Since the P wave represents atrial depolarization, we look at the P wave to assess atrial enlargement. Similarly, we examine the QRS complex to determine if there is ventricular hypertrophy.

---

* More recently, the term atrial enlargement has been supplanted in the minds of some by the term *atrial abnormalities*. This change in terminology reflects the recognition that a variety of electrical abnormalities can cause the changes on the EKG characteristically associated with atrial enlargement. However, we will continue to use the term "atrial enlargement" in this book, both because the term is more rooted in tradition (and traditional values still carry some value as we race headlong into the next millenium), and because the vast majority of cases of P wave changes are due to enlargement of the atria.

How the EKG Can Change

Three things can happen to a wave on the EKG when a chamber hypertrophies or enlarges:

1. The chamber may take longer to depolarize. The EKG wave may therefore *increase in duration.*

2. The chamber may generate more current and thus a larger voltage. The wave may therefore *increase in amplitude.*

3. A larger percentage of the total electrical current may move through the expanded chamber. The mean electrical vector, or what we call the *electrical axis,* of the EKG wave may therefore shift.

Because the concept of axis is so important for diagnosing hypertrophy and enlargement, we need to digress for just a moment to elaborate on this concept.

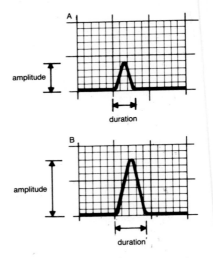

(*A*) A normal wave. (*B*) The same wave when the chamber has enlarged or hypertrophied. The amplitude and duration of the wave have increased. A third alteration, a shift in the electrical axis, will be discussed in the following pages.

Axis

Earlier we discussed how the EKG records the instantaneous vector of electrical forces at any given moment. Using this idea, we can represent the complete depolarization (or repolarization) of a chamber by drawing a series of sequential vectors, each representing the sum of all electrical forces at a given moment.

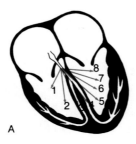

A

Ventricular depolarization is represented by eight sequential instantaneous vectors, illustrating how the electrical forces normally move progressively leftward. Although we have shown only eight instantaneous vectors, we could have shown 18 or 80. We chose eight out of compassion for our artist.

The first vector represents septal depolarization, and each successive vector represents progressive depolarization of the ventricles. The vectors swing progressively leftward because the electrical activity of the much larger left ventricle increasingly dominates the EKG.

The average vector of all of the instantaneous vectors is called the *mean vector.*

The *direction* of the mean vector is called the **mean electrical axis.**

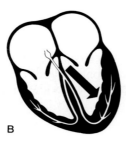

B

A single vector summarizes all of the instantaneous vectors. This summation vector is called the mean vector, and its direction is the axis of ventricular depolarization. Axis is defined in the frontal plane only.

The mean QRS vector points leftward and inferiorly, representing the average direction of current flow during ventricular depolarization. The normal QRS *axis*—the direction of this mean vector—thus lies between +90° and 0°. (Actually, most cardiologists extend the range of normal from +90° to −30°. In time, as you become more comfortable with the concept of axis, you should add this refinement to your electrical analysis, but for now +90° to 0° will be quite satisfactory.)

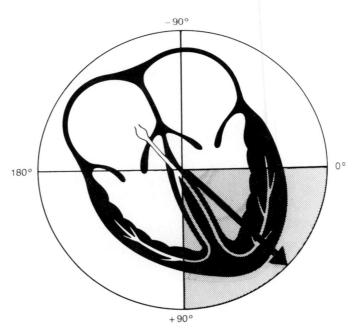

If the QRS axis lies within the shaded quadrant, between 0° and 90°, it is normal.

We can quickly determine whether the QRS axis on any EKG is normal by looking only at leads I and AVF. **If the QRS complex is positive in leads I and AVF, the QRS axis must be normal.**

Why is this?

Determining Whether the QRS Axis Is Normal

We know that any lead will record a positive deflection if the wave of depolarization is moving toward it. Lead I is oriented at 0°. Thus, if the mean QRS vector is directed anywhere between −90° and +90°, lead I will record a predominantly positive QRS complex.

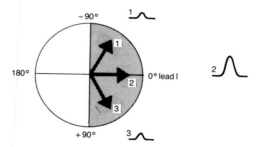

Any mean QRS vector oriented between −90° and +90° will produce a predominantly positive QRS complex in lead I. Three different QRS mean vectors are shown. All three are oriented between −90° and +90°; hence, they will all produce a predominantly positive QRS complex. The three QRS complexes depicted here illustrate what lead I would record for each of the three vectors.

Lead AVF is oriented at +90°. If the mean QRS vector is directed anywhere between 0° and 180°, lead AVF will record a predominantly positive QRS complex.

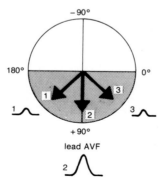

Any mean QRS vector oriented between 0° and 180° will produce a predominantly positive QRS complex in lead AVF. Three different mean QRS vectors are shown, all oriented so that lead AVF will record a predominantly positive deflection as illustrated.

If the QRS complex is predominantly positive in *both* lead I and lead AVF, then the QRS axis must lie between 0° and +90°. This is the normal QRS axis.

Another way to look at this is to take the converse approach: **if the QRS complex in either lead I or lead AVF is *not* predominantly positive, then the QRS axis does *not* lie between 0° and +90°, and it is *not* normal.**

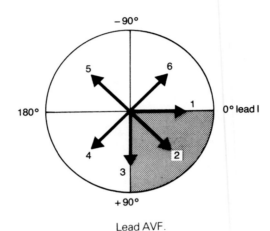

Lead AVF.

	lead I	lead AVF
1	⌐Ⅼ⌐	⌐Ⅴ⌐
2	⌐Ⅼ⌐	⌐Ⅼ⌐
3	⌐Ⅴ⌐	⌐Ⅼ⌐
4	⌐Ⅴ⌐	⌐Ⅼ⌐
5	⌐Ⅴ⌐	⌐Ⅴ⌐
6	⌐Ⅼ⌐	⌐Ⅴ⌐

Six different QRS axes are shown (*A*). Only an axis directed between 0° and +90° *(shaded quadrant)* will produce a predominantly positive QRS complex in both lead I and lead AVF. (*B*) The QRS complexes in leads I and AVF associated with each of the six axes are shown. Only axis 2 is normal and associated with a predominantly positive QRS complex in both leads, although most cardiologists would consider axis 1 and axis 3 to be essentially normal as well.

Defining the Axis Precisely

Although it is usually sufficient to note whether the axis is normal or not, it is possible to be a bit more rigorous and to define the actual angle of the axis with fair precision. All you need to do is look for the limb lead in which the QRS complex is most nearly biphasic, with positive and negative deflections virtually equal (sometimes the deflections are so small that the wave appears flat, or iso-electric). The axis must then be oriented approximately perpendicular to this lead, because an electrode oriented perpendicularly to the mean direction of current flow records a biphasic wave.

Thus, for example, if the QRS complex in lead III (orientation +120°) is biphasic, then the axis must be oriented at right angles (90°) to this lead, either at +30° or −150°. And, if we already know that the axis is normal—that is, if the QRS complex is positive in leads I and AVF—then the axis cannot be −150°, but must be +30°.

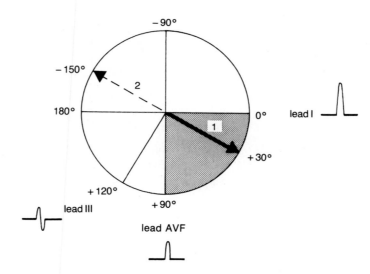

QRS complexes are shown for leads I, III, and AVF. Determining the axis is easy. The QRS complex in lead III is biphasic. The axis therefore must be either +30° or −150°. However, since the QRS complex is positive in both leads I and AVF, the axis must be normal, *i.e.*, it must lie within the shaded quadrant. The axis therefore can be only +30°.

Axis Deviation: Getting More Specific About Defining Abnormal Axes

The normal QRS axis is between 0° and 90°. If the axis lies between 90° and 180°, we speak of *right axis deviation*. Will the QRS complex in leads I and AVF be positive or negative in a patient with right axis deviation?

The QRS complex in lead AVF will still be positive, but it will be negative in lead I.

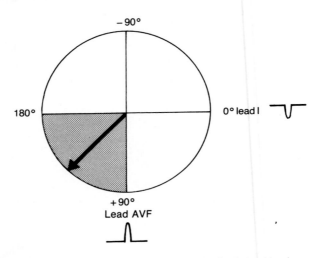

Right axis deviation. The QRS complex is negative in lead I, whereas it is positive in AVF.

If the axis lies between 0° and −90°, we speak of *left axis deviation*. In this case, the QRS complex in lead I will be positive, but it will be negative in lead AVF.

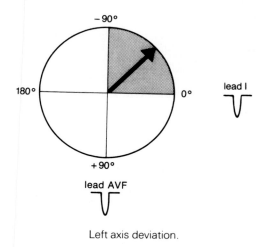

Left axis deviation.

In rare instances, the axis becomes totally disoriented and lies between −90° and 180°. This is called *extreme right axis deviation*. The QRS complex in both lead AVF and lead I will be negative.

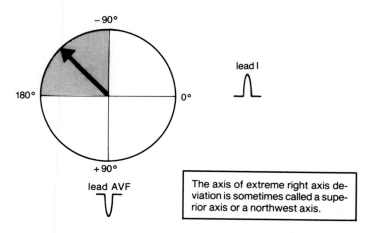

The axis of extreme right axis deviation is sometimes called a superior axis or a northwest axis.

Extreme right axis deviation.

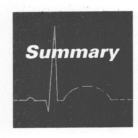

Summary

Axis

1. The term *axis* refers to the direction of the mean electrical vector, representing the average direction of current flow. It is defined in the frontal plane only.

2. To determine the axis, find the lead in which the QRS complex is most nearly biphasic. The QRS axis must lie approximately perpendicular to the axis.

3. A quick estimate of the axis can be made by looking at leads I and AVF:

Axis	Lead I	Lead AVF
Normal axis	Positive	Positive
Left axis deviation	Positive	Negative
Right axis deviation	Negative	Positive
Extreme right axis deviation	Negative	Negative

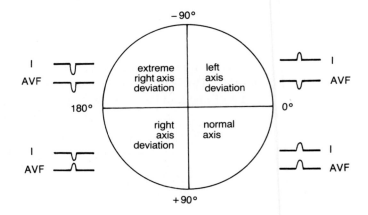

On the EKG below, the waves recorded by the six leads of the frontal plane are shown. Is the QRS axis normal or is there axis deviation?

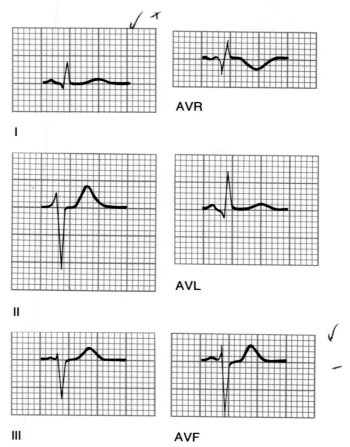

I

AVR

II

AVL

III

AVF

This patient has left axis deviation; the QRS complex is predominantly positive in lead I and negative in lead AVF.

Now, can you define the axis more precisely by finding the lead with a biphasic QRS complex?

The QRS complex in lead AVR is approximately biphasic, so the electrical axis must lie nearly perpendicular to it, *i.e.,* at either −60° or +120°. Because we already know that the axis falls within the zone of left axis deviation, *i.e.,* between 0° and −90°, the correct axis must be −60°.

Just as we have done for the QRS complex, so we can define an axis for the P wave and T wave on every EKG. The normal P wave axis lies between 0° and 75° in adults and between 0° and 90° in children. The T wave axis is variable, but it should lie within 50° to 60° of the QRS axis.

Can you identify the axis of the QRS complex, P wave, and T wave on the following EKG?

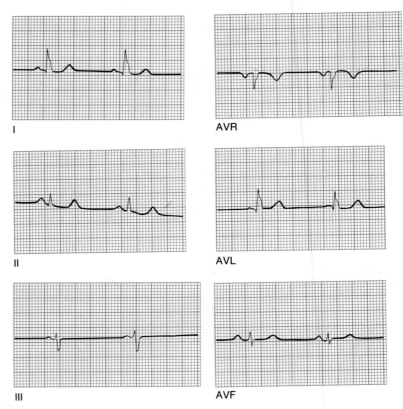

(A) The QRS axis is approximately 0°. It is nearly biphasic in AVF, implying an axis of 0° or 180°. Since the QRS complex in lead I has a tall R wave, the axis must be 0°. (B) Lead II has the most positive P wave. The P wave axis is approximately +60°. (C) All of the leads with tall R waves have positive T waves. The T waves are flat in lead III, indicating an axis perpendicular to lead III (either +30° or −150°). Since there is a tall T wave in lead I, the axis must be approximately +30°.

⊞ *Axis Deviation, Hypertrophy, and Enlargement*

Why does axis deviation have anything to do with hypertrophy and enlargement? Since the concept of axis deviation is most successfully applied to ventricular hypertrophy, let's consider what happens to the flow of electricity when a ventricle hypertrophies.

In the normal heart, the QRS axis lies between 0° and +90°, reflecting the electrical dominance of the much larger left ventricle over the right ventricle. Imagine, now, a 65-year-old male who has allowed his hypertension to go untreated for many years. He comes to see you for headaches and shortness of breath, and you discover a greatly elevated blood pressure of 190/115 mm Hg. This sustained and severe hypertension has forced the left ventricle to work too hard for too long, and it hypertrophies. Its electrical dominance over the right ventricle therefore becomes even more profound. The mean electrical vector is drawn even further leftward, and the result is *left axis deviation.*

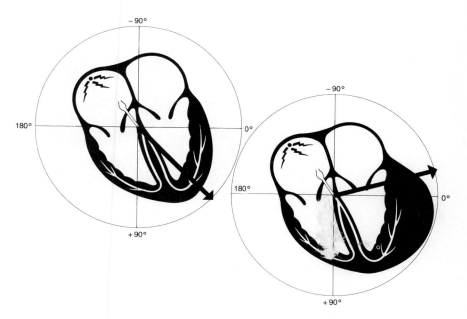

With left ventricular hypertrophy, the electrical axis moves further leftward, resulting in left axis deviation.

Right ventricular hypertrophy is far less common, and requires a huge change in the proportions of the right ventricle in order to overcome the electrical forces generated by the normally dominant left ventricle. It can occur, however, in cases of severe pulmonary stenosis or primary pulmonary hypertension. If the right ventricle hypertrophies sufficiently, it can be detected on the EKG as a shift in the QRS axis. The mean electrical axis of current flow is drawn rightward, and the result is *right axis deviation.*

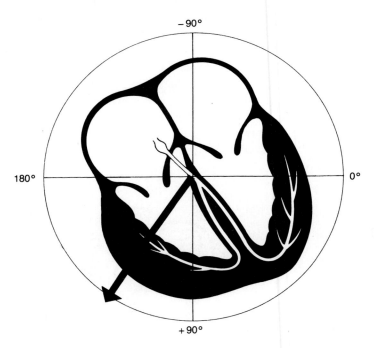

With right ventricular hypertrophy, the electrical axis moves rightward, resulting in right axis deviation.

This is a good time to restate the three things that can happen to a wave on the EKG with enlargement or hypertrophy:

1. The wave can increase in duration.

2. The wave can increase in amplitude.

3. There can be axis deviation.

Specific EKG criteria for the diagnosis of atrial enlargement and ventricular hypertrophy have been devised, and these are discussed in the following pages.

⊞ *Atrial Enlargement*

The normal P wave is less than 0.12 seconds in duration, and the largest deflection, whether positive or negative, should not exceed 2.5 mm. The first part of the P wave represents right atrial depolarization, and the second part left atrial depolarization.

Virtually all of the information you need to assess atrial enlargement can be found in leads II and V_1. Lead II is useful because it is oriented nearly parallel to the flow of current through the atria (*i.e.*, parallel to the mean P wave vector). It therefore records the largest positive deflection and is very sensitive to any perturbations in atrial depolarization. Lead V_1 is useful because it is oriented perpendicularly to the flow of electricity and is therefore biphasic, allowing easy separation of the right and left atrial components.

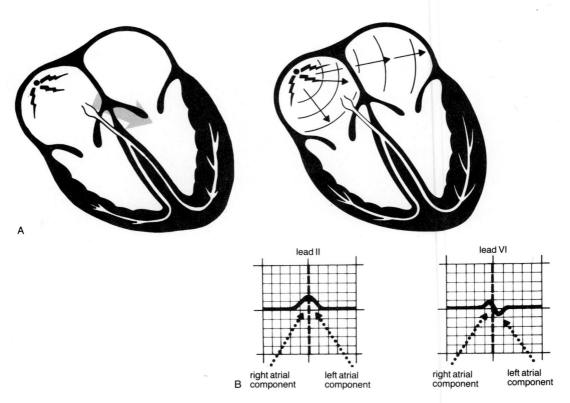

(*A*) Normal atrial depolarization. (*B*) The normal P wave in leads II and V_1. The first part of the P wave represents right atrial depolarization, the second part represents left atrial depolarization.

Right Atrial Enlargement

With *right atrial enlargement,* the amplitude of the first portion of the P wave increases to 3 mm or more. The width does *not* change, because the terminal component of the P wave is the *left* atrial in origin, and this remains unchanged.

Enlargement of the right atrium may also cause the right atrium to dominate the left atrium electrically. The vector of atrial depolarization may swing rightward, and the P wave axis may move rightward +90°. The tallest P wave may therefore no longer appear in lead II, but in lead AVF or lead III.

The classic picture of right atrial enlargement, illustrated in leads II and V₁, below, is called *P pulmonale,* because it is often caused by severe lung disease.

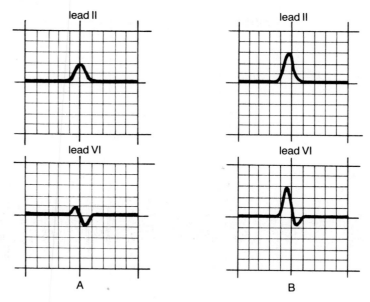

(*A*) The normal P wave in leads II and V₁. (*B*) Right atrial enlargement. Note the increased amplitude of the early, right atrial component of the P wave. The terminal left atrial component, and hence the overall duration of the P wave, is essentially unchanged.

Left Atrial Enlargement

With *left atrial enlargement*, the second portion of the P wave may increase in amplitude. The diagnosis of left atrial enlargement requires that the terminal (left atrial) portion of the P wave should drop at least 1 mm below the isoelectric line.

However, a more prominent change in the P wave is an increase in its *duration*. This occurs because left atrial depolarization represents the terminal portion of the P wave, and prolonged depolarization can be readily seen (with *right* atrial enlargement, prolonged depolarization of the right atrium is hidden by the left atrial portion of the P wave). The diagnosis of left atrial enlargement, therefore, also requires that the terminal portion of the P wave should be at least one small block (0.04 seconds) in width.

The electrocardiographic picture of left atrial enlargement is often called *P mitrale*, because mitral valve disease is a common cause of left atrial enlargement.

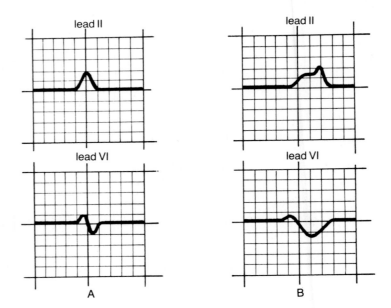

(*A*) Again, the normal P wave in leads II and V$_1$. (*B*) Left atrial enlargement. Note the increased amplitude and duration of the terminal, left atrial component of the P wave.

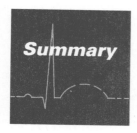

Summary

Atrial Enlargement

To diagnose atrial enlargement, look at leads II and V₁.
Right atrial enlargement is characterized by the following:

1. Increased amplitude of the first portion of the P wave

2. No change in the duration of the P wave

3. Possible right axis deviation of the P wave

Left atrial enlargement is characterized by the following:

1. The amplitude of the terminal (negative) component of the P wave may be increased, and must descend at least 1 mm below the isoelectric line

2. The duration of the P wave is increased, and the terminal (negative) portion of the P wave must be at least 1 small block (0.04 seconds) in width

3. No significant axis deviation is seen, because the left atrium is normally electrically dominant

It should be stressed again that electrocardiographic evidence of atrial enlargement (especially left atrial enlargement) often has no pathologic correlate, and may in some cases merely reflect some nonspecific conduction abnormality. Interpretation of atrial enlargement on the EKG must therefore be tempered by knowledge of the clinical setting (a good idea in any circumstance!).

⊞ *Ventricular Hypertrophy*

The diagnosis of ventricular hypertrophy requires a careful assessment of the QRS complex in many leads.

Right Ventricular Hypertrophy

Looking at the Limb Leads

In the limb leads, the most common feature associated with right ventricular hypertrophy is right axis deviation; *i.e.*, the electrical axis of the QRS complex, normally between 0° and +90°, veers between +90° and +180°. This reflects the new electrical dominance of the usually electrically submissive right ventricle.

Many cardiologists feel that the QRS axis must exceed +100° in order to make the diagnosis of right ventricular hypertrophy. Therefore, the QRS complex in lead I (oriented at 0°) must be slightly more negative than positive.

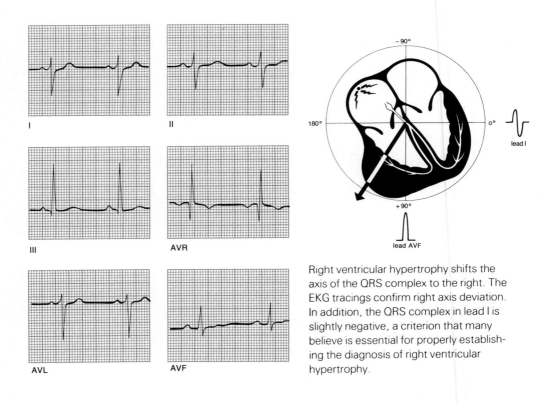

Right ventricular hypertrophy shifts the axis of the QRS complex to the right. The EKG tracings confirm right axis deviation. In addition, the QRS complex in lead I is slightly negative, a criterion that many believe is essential for properly establishing the diagnosis of right ventricular hypertrophy.

Looking at the Precordial Leads

The precordial leads can also be helpful in diagnosing right ventricular hypertrophy. As you might expect, the normal pattern of R wave progression, whereby the R wave amplitude enlarges as you proceed from lead V_1 to V_5, is disrupted. Instead of the R wave amplitude increasing as the leads move closer to the left ventricle, the reverse may occur. There may be a large R wave in lead V_1, which lies over the hypertrophied right ventricle, and a small R wave in lead V_6, which lies over the normal, but now electrically humble, left ventricle. Similarly, the S wave in lead V_1 is small, whereas the S wave in lead V_6 is large.

These criteria have been expressed in simple mathematics:

- In lead V_1, the R wave is larger than the S wave.

- In lead V_6, the S wave is larger than the R wave.

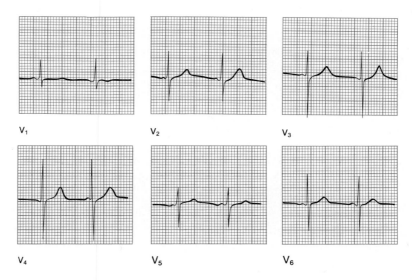

In lead V_1, the R wave is larger than the S wave. In lead V_6, the S wave is larger than the R wave.

The most common causes of right ventricular hypertrophy are pulmonary disease and congenital heart disease.

Left Ventricular Hypertrophy

The diagnosis of left ventricular hypertrophy is somewhat more complicated. Left axis deviation beyond −15° is often seen, but by and large this is not a very useful diagnostic feature. Instead, *increased R wave amplitude over those leads overlying the left ventricle forms the basis for the EKG diagnosis of left ventricular hypertrophy.*

Unfortunately, there are almost as many criteria for diagnosing left ventricular hypertrophy on the EKG as there are books about EKGs. Nevertheless, all the criteria reflect a common theme: **there should be increased R wave amplitude in leads overlying the left ventricle, and increased S wave amplitude in leads overlying the right ventricle.** The criteria listed here are not the only ones, but they will serve you well:

Looking at the Precordial Leads

In general, the precordial leads are more sensitive than the limb leads for the diagnosis of left ventricular hypertrophy. The most useful criteria in the precordial leads are as follows:

1. The R wave amplitude in lead V_5 or V_6 *plus* the S wave amplitude in lead V_1 or V_2 exceeds 35 mm.

2. The R wave amplitude in lead V_5 exceeds 26 mm.

3. The R wave amplitude in lead V_6 exceeds 18 mm.

4. The R wave amplitude in lead V_6 exceeds the R wave amplitude in lead V_5.

The more criteria that are positive, the greater the likelihood that the patient has left ventricular hypertrophy.

It is, sadly, worth your while to memorize all of these criteria, but if you want to be selective, choose the first since it is probably the most accurate.

Note: These criteria are of little value in individuals less than 35 years old who frequently have increased voltage due, in many cases, to a relatively thin chest wall.

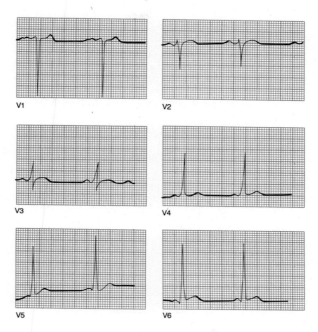

Left ventricular hypertrophy in the precordial leads. Three of the four criteria are met: the R wave amplitude in V_5 plus the S wave amplitude in V_1 exceeds 35 mm, the R wave amplitude in V_6 exceeds 18 mm, and the R wave amplitude in lead V_6 slightly exceeds the R wave amplitude in lead V_5. The only criterion not met is for the R wave in lead V_5 to exceed 26 mm.

Looking at the Limb Leads

The most useful criteria in the limb leads are as follows:

1. The R wave amplitude in lead AVL exceeds 13 mm.

2. The R wave amplitude in lead AVF exceeds 21 mm.

3. The R wave amplitude in lead I exceeds 14 mm.

4. The R wave amplitude in lead I *plus* the S wave amplitude in lead III exceeds 25 mm.

Again, if you aspire to electrocardiographic nirvana, learn them all. If you must pick one, pick the first.

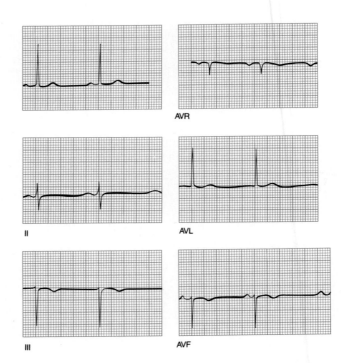

Left ventricular hypertrophy in the limb leads. Criteria 1, 3, and 4 are met; only criterion 2, regarding the R wave amplitude in lead AVF, is not met.

The leading causes of left ventricular hypertrophy are systemic hypertension and valvular disease.

You may have noticed that no comment has been made about the *duration* of the QRS complex. Both right and left ventricular hypertrophy may slightly prolong the QRS complex, but rarely beyond 0.1 seconds.

When Both Ventricles Are Hypertrophied

What happens when *both* the right ventricle and left ventricle are hypertrophied? As you might expect, there may be a combination of features (*e.g.,* left ventricular hypertrophy in the precordial leads with right axis deviation in the limb leads), but in most cases the effects of left ventricular hypertrophy will obscure those of right ventricular hypertrophy.

Is there ventricular hypertrophy in the tracing below?

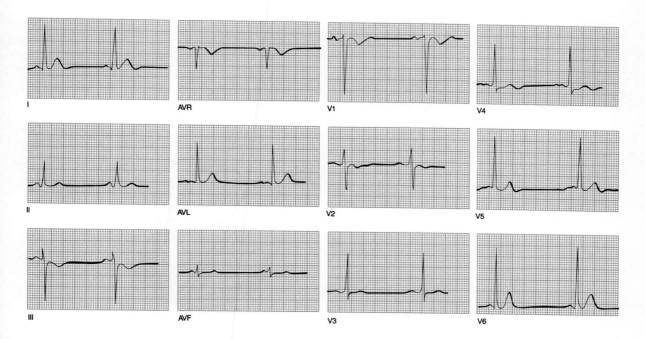

Yes. This patient had aortic stenosis and has left ventricular hypertrophy on the EKG. He meets the criteria in both the precordial and limb leads.

⊞ *Strain*

Something else may happen with severe ventricular hypertrophy. The myocardium can become so thickened that part of it may not get all of the blood supply it needs. The part of the myocardium that is most vulnerable to hypoxia is the subendocardium, the inner layer of the myocardium lying just beneath the endocardial lining of the four chambers. Whereas uncomplicated ventricular hypertrophy causes EKG changes only in the QRS complex, subendocardial ischemia causes changes in the ST segment and T wave. As we shall see in the chapter on myocardial infarction, the ST segment and T wave are very susceptible to the effects of ischemia. Another way to look at this is that uncomplicated ventricular hypertrophy affects ventricular depolarization, whereas ventricular hypertrophy associated with subendocardial ischemia affects both ventricular depolarization and repolarization.

The ST segment and T wave changes that sometimes accompany ventricular hypertrophy are called *strain*. They include

- ST segment depression

- T wave inversion

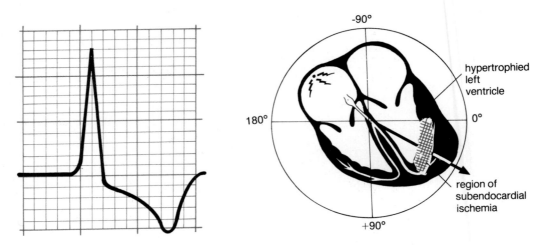

Strain. Note how the depressed ST segment and the inverted T wave seem to blend together to form a single asymmetric wave. The downward slope is gradual; the upward slope is abrupt.

Strain is most evident in those leads with tall R waves (reasonably so, since these leads lie over, and most directly reflect, the electrical forces of the hypertrophied ventricle). Thus, right ventricular strain will be seen in leads V_1 and V_2, and left ventricular strain will be most evident in leads I, AVL, V_5, and V_6.

Strain usually indicates severe hypertrophy and may even herald the onset of ventricular dilatation. For example, a patient with aortic stenosis and no symptoms may show a stable pattern of left ventricular hypertrophy for years. Eventually, however, the left ventricle may fail, and the patient will develop severe shortness of breath and other symptoms of congestive heart failure. The EKG may then show left ventricular hypertrophy with strain. This progression is illustrated in the two EKGs below.

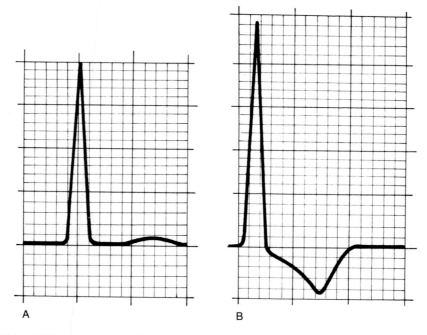

A   B

(A) Lead AVL in a patient with left aortic stenosis and left ventricular hypertrophy. Note the tall R wave, meeting the criteria for left ventricular hypertrophy. The ST segment is flat and the T wave is just barely upright. (B) One year later, the same lead shows the development of a strain pattern, signifying in this case the onset of left ventricular failure. The ST segment is depressed and the T wave inverted. Note, too, that the R wave has become even taller.

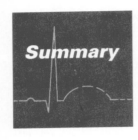

Summary

Ventricular Hypertrophy

Right ventricular hypertrophy is characterized by the following:

1. Right axis deviation is present, with the QRS axis exceeding +100°.

2. The R wave is larger than the S wave in V_1, whereas the S wave is larger than the R wave in V_6.

Left ventricular hypertrophy is characterized by many criteria. The two most useful are the following:

1. The R wave in V_5 or V_6 plus the S wave in V_1 or V_2 exceeds 35 mm.

2. The R wave in AVL exceeds 13 mm.

The presence of *strain* is diagnosed on the EKG by finding asymmetric ST segment depression and T inversion, most often in leads with tall R waves. Strain indicates clinically significant hypertrophy and may herald the development of ventricular dilatation and failure.

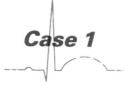

Case 1

Mildred W., a 53-year-old widow (her husband died of cerebral anoxia induced by his futile efforts to memorize all of the EKG criteria for left ventricular hypertrophy), comes to your office for a routine checkup. She is new to your practice and has not seen a doctor since her last child was born, which was over 20 years ago. She has no specific complaints besides an occasional sinus headache. Routine physical examination is unremarkable, except that you find that her blood pressure is 170/110. She is unaware of being hypertensive. You would like to know if her hypertension is long-standing or of recent onset. Your laboratory assessment includes serum electrolytes, creatinine, blood urea nitrogen, urinalysis, chest x-ray, and the EKG shown below. Is the EKG helpful?

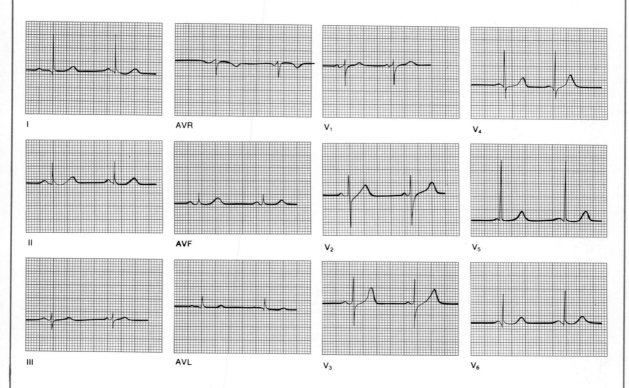

Mildred's EKG is essentially normal, which is not at all surprising. Most patients with hypertension have normal cardiograms. Nevertheless, had you found left ventricular hypertrophy, with or without strain, you would have had at least one piece of evidence suggesting that her hypertension is long-standing.

Case 2

Tom L. is a 23-year-old marathon runner. Topping Heartbreak Hill at about the 20-mile mark of the Boston Marathon, he suddenly turns pale, clutches his chest, and drops to the ground. Another runner, although right on pace for a personal best, stops to help. Finding Tom pulseless and apneic, he begins cardiopulmonary resuscitation. The timely intervention proves life-saving. Tom responds, and moments later the following EKG is taken as he is being rushed to the nearest hospital. Why did Tom collapse?

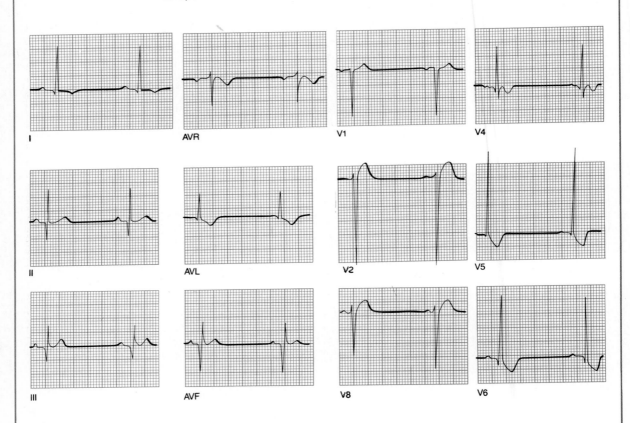

Hint: If you get this, you already know too much.

Tom L. collapsed because of a hypertrophic disease of his heart muscle. A leading cause of sudden death in young, healthy athletes is hypertrophic cardiomyopathy, of which one variant is called *idiopathic hypertrophic subaortic stenosis,* or *IHSS* (it is also called asymmetric septal hypertrophy). In this disorder, the ventricles and the interventricular septum can become grossly hypertrophied. In many cases it is hereditary, and the resultant clinical repercussions can range from severe and life-threatening to virtually nothing at all. Death can result from (1) obstruction to left ventricular outflow by the hypertrophied muscle; (2) impaired filling of the stiff, hypertrophied left ventricle during diastole; or (3) a cardiac arrhythmia. The classic features on the EKG are

1. Ventricular hypertrophy

2. Strain patterns in those leads with the tallest R waves

3. Q waves, of uncertain etiology, in the inferior and lateral leads

Although this case was patently unfair, you may have recognized some of the features we have been talking about in this chapter, namely the presence of criteria for left ventricular hypertrophy, especially in the precordial leads. Strain is evident in all the left lateral leads (I, AVL, V_5, and V_6). Note, too, the deep Q waves in leads II, III, and AVF, typical of this disorder.

The timely intervention of his fellow runner saved Tom's life. It turned out that he had had similar, albeit less severe, episodes in the past, characterized by lightheadedness and chest pain. He was subsequently placed on verapamil, a calcium channel blocker, which prevented any recurrence of his symptoms. Verapamil reduces myocardial oxygen consumption, thereby preventing ischemia of the hypertrophied muscle, and improves the compliance of the stiffened ventricle. Beta blockers are also used in this condition; they too lessen the risk of significant ischemia and may also prevent arrhythmias.

The Only EKG Book You'll Ever Need, second edition, by Malcolm S. Thaler.
JB Lippincott Company, Philadelphia © 1995.

3 Arrhythmias

In this chapter you will learn:

1 what an arrhythmia is, and what it does (and doesn't do) to people

2 about rhythm strips, Holter monitors, and event monitors

3 to determine the heart rate from the EKG

4 the four basic types of arrhythmias

5 to recognize the four common types of sinus arrhythmias

6 what an ectopic rhythm is, and the mechanisms of its formation

7 to ask The Four Questions that will let you recognize and diagnose the common ectopic arrhythmias that originate in the atria, the AV node, and the ventricles

8 to distinguish supraventricular arrhythmias from ventricular arrhythmias, both clinically and on the EKG

9 how Programmed Electrical Stimulation and other new techniques have revolutionized the diagnosis and treatment of certain arrhythmias

10 about the cases of Lola deB. and George M., with which you will astonish yourself with how easily you have mastered material that has cowed the high and mighty.

The heart normally beats with a regular rhythm, 60 to 100 times per minute. Because each beat originates with depolarization of the sinus node, the usual, everyday cardiac rhythm is called *normal sinus rhythm*. Anything else is called an *arrhythmia* (or, perhaps more accurately, a *dysrhythmia,* but again we shall opt for the more conventional term in the discussion to follow).

The term *arrhythmia* refers to any disturbance in the rate, regularity, site of origin, or conduction of the cardiac electrical impulse. An arrhythmia can be a single aberrant beat (or even a prolonged pause between beats) or a sustained rhythm disturbance that can persist for the lifetime of the patient.

Not every arrhythmia is abnormal or dangerous. For example, heart rates as low as 40 beats per minute are common and quite normal in well-trained athletes. Single abnormal beats, originating elsewhere in the heart than the sinus node, frequently occur in the majority of healthy individuals.

Many arrhythmias, however, can be dangerous, and some require immediate therapy to prevent sudden death. The diagnosis of an arrhythmia is one of the most important things an EKG can do, and nothing yet has been found that can do it better.

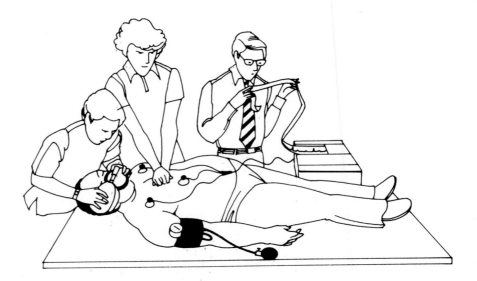

⊞ *The Clinical Manifestations of Arrhythmias*

When should you suspect that someone had or is having an arrhythmia?

Many arrhythmias go unnoticed by the patient and are picked up incidentally on a routine physical examination or EKG. Frequently, however, arrhythmias elicit one of several characteristic symptoms.

First and foremost are *palpitations,* an awareness of one's own heartbeat. Patients may describe intermittent accelerations or decelerations of their heartbeat, or a sustained rapid heartbeat that may be regular or irregular. The sensation may be no more than a mild nuisance or a truly terrifying experience.

More serious are symptoms of decreased cardiac output, which can occur when the arrhythmia compromises cardiac function. Among these are *lightheadedness* and *syncope* (a sudden faint).

Rapid arrhythmias can increase the oxygen demands of the myocardium and cause *angina* (chest pain). The sudden onset of an arrhythmia in a patient with underlying cardiac disease can also precipitate *congestive heart failure.*

Sometimes the first clinical manifestation of an arrhythmia is *sudden death.* Patients in the throes of an acute myocardial infarction are at a greatly increased risk of arrhythmic sudden death, which is why they are hospitalized in cardiac care units where their heart rate and rhythm can be continuously monitored. Because arrhythmias are so common in this setting, it is the policy of some hospitals to treat all of their heart attack patients with antirrhythmic drugs *prophylactically,* even if there is no evidence of an arrhythmia on the cardiac monitor.

⊞ *Why Arrhythmias Happen*

It is often impossible to identify the underlying cause of an arrhythmia, but a careful search for treatable precipitating factors must always be made. The mnemonic HIS DEBS, here offered in print for the first (and possibly last) time, should help you remember those arrhythmogenic factors that should be considered whenever you encounter a patient with an arrhythmia.

H—Hypoxia: A myocardium deprived of oxygen is an irritable myocardium. Pulmonary disorders, whether severe chronic lung disease or an acute pulmonary embolus, are major precipitants of cardiac arrhythmias.

I—Ischemia: We have already mentioned that myocardial infarctions are a common setting for arrhythmias. Angina, even without the actual death of myocardial cells associated with infarction, is also a major precipitant.

S—Sympathetic Stimulation: Enhanced sympathetic tone from any cause (hyperthyroidism, congestive heart failure, nervousness, exercise, etc.) can elicit arrhythmias.

D—Drugs: Many drugs can cause arrhythmias. Ironically, the antiarrhythmic drugs themselves, such as quinidine, are among the leading culprits.

E—Electrolyte Disturbances: Hypokalemia is notorious for its ability to induce arrhythmias, but imbalances of calcium and magnesium can also be responsible.

B—Bradycardia: A very slow heart rate seems to predispose one to arrhythmias. One could include the brady-tachy syndrome (also called the sick sinus syndrome) in this category.

S—Stretch: Enlargement and hypertrophy of the atria and ventricles can produce arrhythmias. This is one way in which congestive heart failure and valvular disease can cause arrhythmias.

⊞ *Rhythm Strips*

In order to identify an arrhythmia correctly, it is often necessary to view the heart rhythm over a much longer period of time than the few complexes present on the standard 12-lead EKG. When an arrhythmia is suspected, either clinically or electrocardiographically, it is standard practice to run a *rhythm strip,* a long tracing of a single lead. Any lead can be chosen, but it obviously makes sense to choose the lead that provides you with the most information. The rhythm strip makes it much easier to identify any rhythmic irregularities or intermittent bursts of unusual electrical activity.

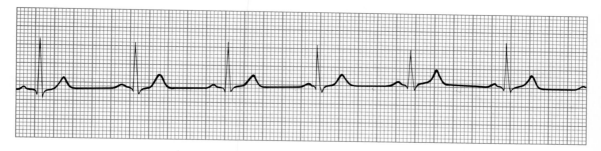

A typical rhythm strip. It can be as short or as long as you need to decipher the rhythm. This particular strip represents a continuous recording of lead II in a patient with normal sinus rhythm, the normal rhythm of the heart.

Holter Monitors and Event Monitors

The ultimate rhythm strip is provided by the *Holter monitor,* or *ambulatory monitor.* The Holter monitor is essentially a portable EKG machine with a memory. The patient wears it for 24 to 48 hours, and a complete record of the patient's heart rhythm is stored and later analyzed for any arrhythmic activity. The monitor can employ one or, more often, two leads (one precordial lead and one limb lead).

Holter monitoring is especially valuable when the suspected arrhythmia is an infrequent occurrence and is therefore unlikely to be captured on a random 12-lead EKG. Clearly, the longer one can monitor the patient, the better the chance that the arrhythmia will be detected. Further information can be obtained if the patient is instructed to write down the precise times when he or she experiences any symptoms. The patient's diary can then be compared with the Holter recording to determine if there is a correlation between the patient's symptoms and any underlying cardiac arrhythmia.

Some rhythm disturbances or symptoms suspicious for arrhythmias happen so infrequently that even a Holter monitor is likely to miss them. For these patients, an *event monitor* may provide a solution. An event monitor records only three to five minutes of a rhythm strip, but it is initiated by the patient when he or she experiences palpitations. The resultant EKG recording is sent out over the phone lines for evaluation. In this manner, multiple recordings can be made over the course of the several months during which the patient has rented the monitor.

How To Determine the Heart Rate From the EKG

The first step in determining the heart's rhythm is to determine the heart rate. It is easily calculated from the EKG.

The horizontal axis on an EKG represents time. The distance between each light line (one small square or 1 mm) equals 0.04 seconds, and the distance between each heavy line (one large square or 5 mm) equals 0.2 seconds. Five large squares therefore constitute 1 second. A cycle that repeats itself every five large squares represents one beat per second, or a heart rate of 60 beats per minute.

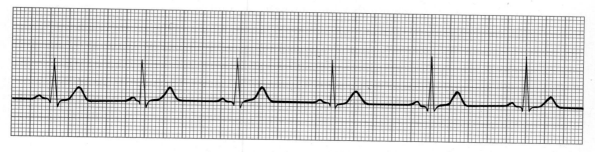

Every QRS complex is separated by five large squares (1 second). A rhythm occurring once every second occurs 60 times every minute.

A Simple Three-Step Method for Calculating the Heart Rate

1. Find an R wave that falls on, or nearly on, one of the heavy lines.

2. Count the number of large squares until the next R wave.

3. Determine the rate in beats per minute as follows:

    - If there is one large square between successive R waves, then each R wave is separated by 0.2 seconds. Therefore, over the course of 1 full second, there will be 5 cycles of cardiac activity (1 second divided by 0.2 seconds), and over 1 minute, 300 cycles (5 × 60 seconds). The heart rate is therefore 300 beats per minute.

    - If there are two large squares between successive R waves, then each R wave is separated by 0.4 seconds. Therefore, over the course of 1 full second, there will be 2.5 cycles of cardiac activity (1 second divided by 0.4 seconds), and over 1 minute, 150 cycles (2.5 × 60 seconds). The heart rate is therefore 150 beats per minute.

By similar logic:

- 3 large squares = 100 beats per minute

- 4 large squares = 75 beats per minute

- 5 large squares = 60 beats per minute

- 6 large squares = 50 beats per minute

Notice that you can get the same answers by dividing 300 by the number of large squares between R waves (*e.g.*, 300 ÷ 4 squares = 75). Even greater accuracy can be achieved by counting the total number of *small* squares between R waves and dividing 1500 by this total.

What is the heart rate on the following strips?

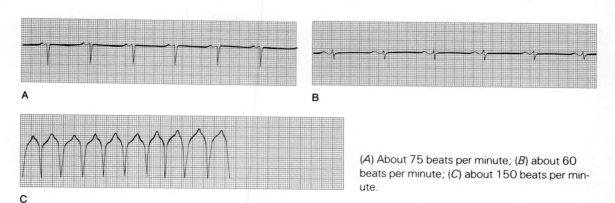

A

B

C

(A) About 75 beats per minute; (B) about 60 beats per minute; (C) about 150 beats per minute.

If the second R wave falls *between* heavy lines, you can estimate that the rate falls between the two extremes on either side.

What is the rate of the following strip?

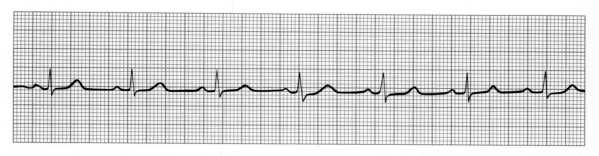

The R waves are slightly more than four squares apart—let's say 4 ¼. The rate must therefore be between 60 and 75 beats per minute. If you guess 70, you'll be close. Alternatively, divide 300 by four and one quarter and get 70.6 beats per minute.

If the heart rate is very slow, you can still use this system; simply divide 300 by the number of large squares between complexes to get your answer. However, there is another method that some prefer. Every EKG strip is marked at 3-second intervals, usually with a series of little lines (or slashes or dots) at the top or bottom of the strip. Count the number of cycles within two of these intervals (6 seconds) and multiply by 10 (10 × 6 seconds = 60 seconds) to get the heart rate in beats per minute. Try it both ways on the example below:

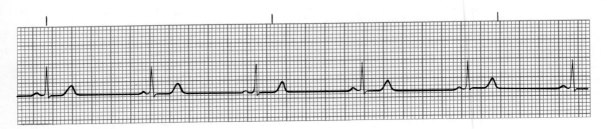

There are approximately four cycles within two of the three second intervals. The rate is therefore about 40 beats per minute (actual rate is 43 beats per minute).

⊞ *The Four Basic Types of Arrhythmias*

Of all of the subjects in electrocardiography, none is guaranteed to cause more anxiety (and palpitations) than the study of arrhythmias. There is no reason for this. First, once you have learned to recognize the basic patterns, nothing is easier than recognizing a classic arrhythmia. Second, the difficult arrhythmias are difficult for everyone, including expert electrocardiographers. Sometimes, in fact, it is impossible to identify what a particular rhythm is. Nothing gladdens one's heart more than the sight of two venerable cardiologists going at it over an insoluble rhythm disturbance.

The heart is capable of only four basic types of rhythm disturbances:

1. The electrical activity follows the usual conduction pathways we have already outlined, but it is either too fast, too slow, or irregular. These are *arrhythmias of sinus origin*.

2. The electrical activity originates elsewhere than the sinus node. These are called *ectopic rhythms*.

3. The electrical activity originates in the sinus node and follows the usual pathways, but encounters unexpected blocks and delays. These *conduction blocks* will be discussed in Chapter 4.

4. The electrical activity follows accessory conduction pathways that bypass the normal ones, providing an electrical shortcut, or short circuit. These arrhythmias are termed *preexcitation syndromes,* and they will be discussed in Chapter 5.

⊞ *Arrhythmias of Sinus Origin*

Sinus Tachycardia and Sinus Bradycardia

Normal sinus rhythm is the normal rhythm of the heart. Depolarization originates spontaneously within the sinus node. The rate is regular and between 60 and 100 beats per minute. If the rhythm speeds up beyond 100, it is called *sinus tachycardia;* if it slows down below 60, it is called *sinus bradycardia.*

Sinus tachycardia and sinus bradycardia can be normal or pathologic. Strenuous exercise, for example, will speed the heart rate over 100 beats per minute, whereas resting heart rates below 60 beats per minute are typical in well-conditioned athletes. On the other hand, alterations in the rate at which the sinus node fires can accompany significant heart disease. Sinus tachycardia can occur in patients with congestive heart failure or severe lung disease, or can be the only presenting sign of hyperthyroidism. Sinus bradycardia is the most common rhythm disturbance seen in the early stages of an acute myocardial infarction; in otherwise healthy individuals, it can result from enhanced vagal tone and can cause fainting.

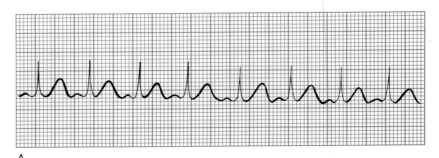

A

B

(*A*) Sinus tachycardia. Each beat is separated by 2 ½ large squares for a rate of 120 beats per minute. (*B*) Sinus bradycardia. More than seven large squares separate each beat, and the rate is 40 to 45 beats per minute.

Sinus Arrhythmia

Often the EKG will reveal a rhythm that appears in all respects to be normal sinus rhythm except that it is slightly irregular. This is called *sinus arrhythmia*. Most often it is a normal phenomenon, reflecting the variation in heart rate with inspiration and expiration. Inspiration accelerates the heart rate, and expiration slows it down.

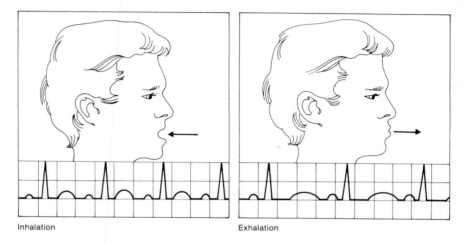

Inhalation

Exhalation

Sinus arrhythmia. The heart rate accelerates with inspiration and slows with expiration.

Sinus Arrest, Asystole, and Escape Beats

Sinus arrest occurs when the sinus node stops firing. If nothing else were to happen, the EKG would show a flat line without any electrical activity, and the patient would die. Prolonged electrical inactivity is called *asystole*.

Fortunately, the heart has pacemaker cells other than the sinus node scattered throughout the myocardium. Ordinarily, the fastest pacemaker drives the heart, and under normal circumstances, the fastest pacemaker is the sinus node. The sinus node *overdrives* the other pacemaker cells by delivering its wave of depolarization throughout the myocardium before its potential competitors can complete their own, more leisurely, spontaneous depolarization. With sinus arrest, however, these other pacemakers can spring into action in a kind of rescue mission. These rescuing beats, originating outside the sinus node, are called *escape beats*.

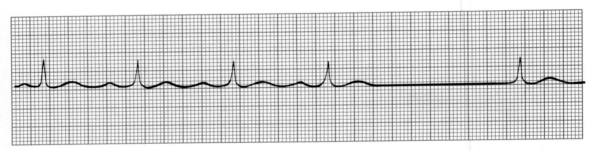

Sinus arrest occurs after the fourth beat. The fifth beat, restoring electrical activity to the heart, is a junctional escape beat.

Nonsinus Pacemakers

Like the sinus node, which typically fires between 60 and 100 times each minute, these other pacemaker cells have their own intrinsic rhythm. *Atrial pacemakers* can discharge at a rate of 60 to 75 beats per minute. Pacemaker cells located near the AV node, called *junctional pacemakers*, can discharge at 40 to 60 beats per minute. *Ventricular pacemaker* cells can discharge at 30 to 45 beats per minute.

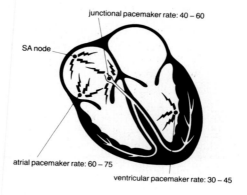

Each of these nonsinus pacemakers can rescue an inadequate sinus node by providing just one or a continual series of escape beats. Of all of the available escape mechanisms, *junctional escape* is by far the most common.

With junctional escape, depolarization originates near the AV node, and the usual pattern of atrial depolarization does not occur. As a result, a normal P wave is not seen. Most often there is no P wave at all. Occasionally, however, a *retrograde P wave* may be seen, representing atrial depolarization moving backward from the AV node into the atria. The mean electrical axis of this retrograde P wave is reversed 180° from that of the normal P wave. Thus, whereas the normal P wave is upright in lead II and inverted in lead AVR, the retrograde P wave is inverted in lead II and upright in lead AVR.

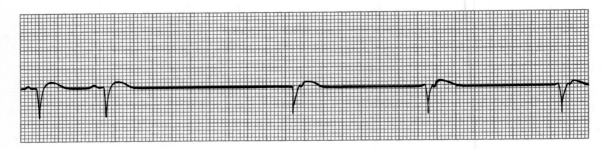

Junctional escape. The first two beats are normal sinus beats with a normal P wave preceding each QRS complex. There is then a long pause followed by a series of three junctional escape beats occurring at a rate of 40 to 45 beats per minute. Retrograde P waves can be seen buried in the T waves. Retrograde P waves can occur before, after, or during the QRS complex, depending on the relative timing of atrial and ventricular depolarization. If atrial and ventricular depolarization occur simultaneously, the much larger QRS complexes will mask the retrograde P waves.

Sinus Arrest Versus Sinus Exit Block

Because sinus node depolarization is *not* recorded on the EKG, it is impossible to determine whether a prolonged sinus pause is due to sinus arrest or to failure of the sinus depolarization to be transmitted out of the node and into the atria, a situation called *sinus exit block*. You may hear these different terms bandied about from time to time, but for all intents and purposes sinus arrest and sinus exit block mean the same thing: there is a failure of the sinus mechanism to deliver its current into the surrounding tissue.

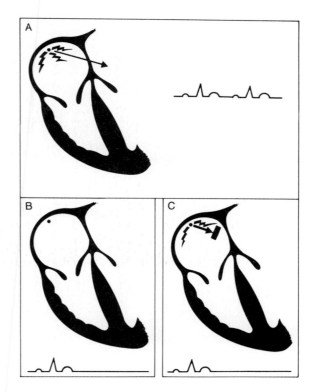

(*A*) Normal sinus rhythm. The sinus node fires repeatedly, and waves of depolarization spread out into the atria. (*B*) Sinus arrest. The sinus node falls silent. No current is generated and the EKG shows no electrical activity. (*C*) Sinus exit block. The sinus node continues to fire, but the wave of depolarization is blocked immediately as it exits the node. Again, the EKG shows no electrical activity.

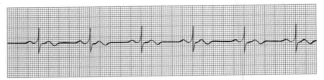

Normal sinus rhythm

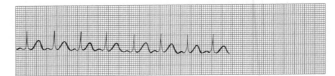

Sinus tachycardia

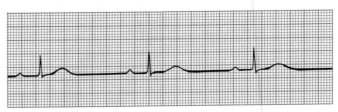

Sinus bradycardia

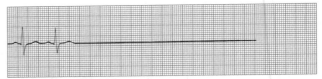

Sinus arrest or exit block

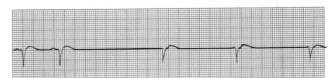

Sinus arrest or exit block with junctional escape

Special note for the electrically infatuated: transient sinus arrest and sinus exit block can sometimes be distinguished on the EKG. With sinus arrest, resumption of sinus electrical activity occurs at any random time (the sinus node simply resumes firing); with sinus exit block, the sinus node has continued to fire silently, and termination of the block allows the sinus node to resume depolarizing the atria after a pause that is some multiple of the normal cycle (exactly one missed P wave, or exactly two missed P waves, or more).

⊞ *Ectopic Rhythms*

Ectopic rhythms are arguably the most important of all of the arrhythmias and the most satisfying to diagnose, because effective therapy is often available.

Ectopic rhythms are abnormal rhythms that arise from elsewhere than the sinus node. In this way they resemble escape beats, but here we are talking about *sustained* rhythms, not just one or a few beats. Ectopic rhythms can be caused by any of the precipitating factors described previously. If we look at the cellular level, there are two physiologic mechanisms by which they can arise: enhanced automaticity and reentry.

Enhanced Automaticity. The fastest pacemaker usually drives the heart, and under normal circumstances the fastest pacemaker is the sinus node. Under *abnormal* circumstances, any of the other pacemakers scattered throughout the heart can be accelerated, *i.e.*, stimulated to depolarize faster and faster until they can overdrive the normal sinus mechanism and establish their own transient or sustained ectopic rhythm. One of the most common causes of enhanced automaticity is digitalis toxicity.

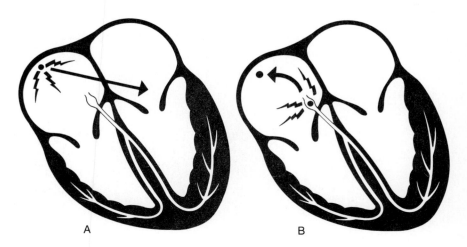

(*A*) Normally, the sinus node drives the heart. (*B*) If another potential pacemaker (*e.g.* the AV junction) is accelerated, it can take over the heart and overdrive the sinus node.

Reentry. Whereas enhanced automaticity represents a disorder of *impulse formation* (*i.e.*, new impulses formed elsewhere than the sinus node take over the heart), reentry represents a disorder of *impulse transmission*. The results, however, are similar: creation of a focus of abnormal electrical activity. Here is how reentry works:

Picture a wave of depolarization arriving at two adjacent regions of myocardium, *A* and *B*, as shown in part *1* of the figure on the next page. *A* and *B* conduct the current at the same rate, and the wave of depolarization rushes past, unperturbed, on its way to new destinations. This is the way things usually operate.

Suppose, however, that pathway *B* transmits the wave of depolarization more slowly than pathway *A*. This could result, for example, if pathway *B* has been damaged by ischemic disease or fibrosis, or if the two pathways are receiving different degrees of input from the autonomic nervous system. This situation is depicted in part *2* of the figure. The wave of depolarization now rushes through pathway *A* but is held up in pathway *B*. The impulse emerging from pathway *A* can now return back through pathway *B*, setting up an uninterrupted revolving circuit along the two pathways (see figure, part *3*). As the electrical impulse spins in this loop, waves of depolarization are sent out in all directions. This is called a *reentry loop*, and it behaves like an electrical generator, providing a source of electrical current that can overdrive the sinus mechanism and run the heart.

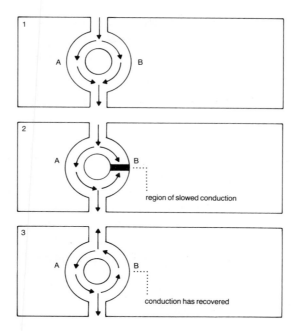

A model showing how a reentrant circuit becomes established. *(1)* Normally pathways *A* and *B* (any two adjacent regions of cardiac function) conduct current equally well. *(2)* Here, however, conduction through pathway *B* is temporarily slowed. Current passing down *A* can then turn back and conduct in a retrograde fashion through *B*. *(3)* The reentry loop is established.

A reentry loop can vary greatly in size. It can be limited to a small loop within a single anatomic site (*e.g.* the AV node), it can loop through an entire chamber (either an atrium or ventricle), or it can even involve both an atrium and ventricle if there is an accessory pathway of conduction connecting the two chambers (this last point will be made more obvious in Chapter 5).

⊞ *The Four Questions*

In order to identify an ectopic rhythm, you need to answer four questions.

Are P Waves Present? If the answer is yes, then the origin of the arrhythmia must be within the atria (an exception to this is the presence of retrograde P waves, which we will discuss later in this chapter). If P waves are not present, then the rhythm must have originated in the AV node or the ventricles.

Are the QRS Complexes Narrow (less than 0.12 seconds in duration) or Wide (greater than 0.12 seconds in duration)? A narrow normal QRS complex implies that ventricular depolarization is proceeding along the usual pathways (AV node to His bundle to bundle branches to Purkinje cells). This is the most efficient means of conduction, requiring the least amount of time, so that the QRS complex is of short duration (narrow). A narrow QRS complex therefore indicates that the origin of the rhythm must be at or above the AV node.

A wide QRS complex usually implies that the origin of ventricular depolarization is within the ventricles themselves. Depolarization is initiated within the ventricular myocardium, not the conduction system, and therefore spreads much more slowly. Conduction does *not* follow the most efficient pathway, and the QRS complex is of long duration (wide).

(The distinction between wide and narrow QRS complexes, although very useful, cannot, unfortunately, be fully relied on to assess the origin of an arrhythmia. We'll see why shortly.)

Questions 1 and 2 thus help to make the important distinction of whether an arrhythmia is ventricular or supraventricular (atrial or junctional) in origin.

What is the Relationship Between the P Waves and the QRS Complexes? If the P wave and QRS complexes correlate in the usual one-to-one fashion, with a single P wave preceding each QRS complex, then the rhythm almost certainly has an atrial origin. Sometimes, however, the atria and ventricles depolarize and contract independently of each other. This will be manifested on the EKG by a lack of correlation between the P waves and QRS complexes, a situation termed *AV dissociation.*

Is the Rhythm Regular or Irregular? This is often the most immediately obvious characteristic of a particular rhythm, and sometimes the most critical.

Whenever you look at an EKG, you will need to assess the rhythm. These four questions should become an intrinsic part of your thinking:

1. Are P waves present?

2. Are the QRS complexes narrow or wide?

3. What is the relationship between the P waves and the QRS complexes?

4. Is the rhythm regular or irregular?

For the normal EKG, the answers are easy:

1. Yes, there are P waves.

2. The QRS complexes are narrow.

3. There is one P wave for every QRS complex.

4. The rhythm is essentially regular.

We will now see what happens when the answers are different.

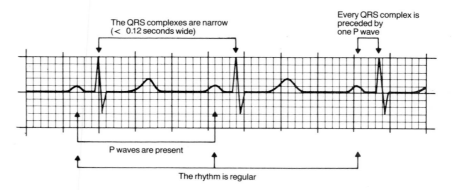

Normal sinus rhythm and "The Four Questions" answered.

⊞ *Ectopic Supraventricular Arrhythmias*

Let us look first at those ectopic arrhythmias that originate in the atria or the AV node, the **supraventricular arrhythmias.**

Atrial arrhythmias can consist of a single beat or a sustained rhythm disturbance lasting for a few seconds or a few years.

Atrial and Junctional Premature Beats

Single ectopic supraventricular beats can originate in the atria or in the vicinity of the AV node. The former are called *atrial premature beats* (or premature atrial contractions); the latter, *junctional premature beats.* These are common phenomena, neither indicating underlying cardiac disease nor requiring treatment. They can, however, initiate more sustained arrhythmias.

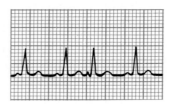

A

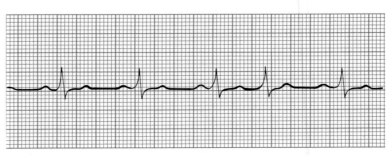

B

(*A*) The third beat is an atrial premature beat. Note how the P wave contour of the premature beat differs from that of the normal sinus beat. (*B*) The fourth beat is a junctional premature beat. There is no P wave preceding the premature QRS complex.

An atrial premature beat can be distinguished from a normal sinus beat by the *contour* of the P wave and by the *timing* of the beat.

Contour. Because an atrial premature beat originates at an atrial site distant from the sinus node, atrial depolarization does not occur in the usual manner and the configuration of the resultant P wave differs from that of the sinus P waves. If the site of origin of the atrial premature beat is far from the sinus node, the *axis* of the atrial premature beat will also differ from that of the normal P waves.

Timing. An atrial premature beat comes too early, *i.e.*, it intrudes itself before the next anticipated sinus wave.

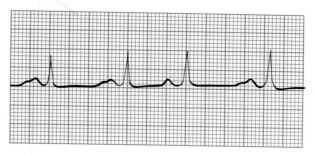

The third beat is an atrial premature beat. The P wave is shaped differently from the other, somewhat unusual-looking P waves, and the beat is clearly premature.

With junctional premature beats, there is usually no visible P wave, but sometimes a retrograde P wave may be seen. This is just like the case with the junctional escape beats seen with sinus arrest.

What is the difference between a junctional premature beat and a junctional escape beat? They look exactly alike, but the junctional premature beat occurs early, prematurely, interposing itself into the normal sinus rhythm. An escape beat occurs late, following a long pause when the sinus node has failed to fire.

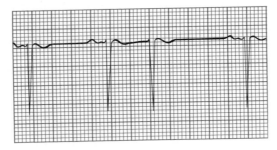

A

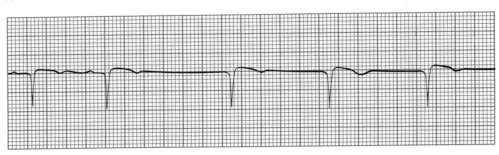

B

(A) A junctional premature beat. The third beat is obviously premature, and there is no P wave preceding the QRS complex. (B) The third beat is a junctional escape beat, establishing a sustained junctional rhythm. It looks just like a junctional premature beat, but it occurs late, following a prolonged pause, rather than prematurely.

Both atrial and junctional premature beats are conducted normally to the ventricles, and the resultant QRS complex is therefore narrow.

There are five types of *sustained* supraventricular arrhythmias that you must learn to recognize:

1. Paroxysmal supraventricular tachycardia (PSVT), sometimes also called AV nodal reentrant tachycardia

2. Atrial flutter

3. Atrial fibrillation

4. Multifocal atrial tachycardia (MAT)

5. Paroxysmal atrial tachycardia (PAT), sometimes also called ectopic atrial tachycardia.

Paroxysmal Supraventricular Tachycardia

Paroxysmal supraventricular tachycardia (PSVT) is a very common arrhythmia. Its onset is sudden, usually initiated by a premature supraventricular beat (atrial or junctional), and its termination is just as abrupt. It can occur in perfectly normal hearts; there may be no underlying cardiac disease at all. Not uncommonly, alcohol, coffee, or just sheer excitement can elicit this rhythm disturbance.

PSVT is an *absolutely regular rhythm,* with a rate usually between 150 and 250 beats per minute. It is driven by a reentrant circuit looping within the AV node. Retrograde P waves may sometimes be seen (your best bet is to look at leads II and III), but more often than not the P waves are buried in the QRS complexes and cannot be identified with any confidence. As with all supraventricular arrhythmias, the QRS complex is narrow.

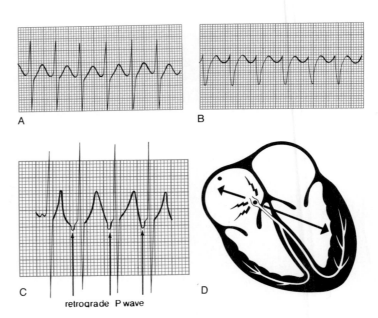

(*A* through *C*) Paroxysmal supraventricular tachycardia in three different patients. Retrograde P waves can be seen just after T waves in *C*. (*D*) The AV node is the site of the reentrant circuit that causes the arrhythmia. Atrial depolarization therefore occurs in reverse, and if P waves can be seen, their axis will be shifted nearly 180° from normal (retrograde P waves).

Carotid Massage

Massaging the carotid artery can help to diagnose and terminate an episode of PSVT. Baroreceptors that sense changes in the blood pressure are located at the angle of the jaw where the common carotid artery bifurcates. When the blood pressure rises, these baroreceptors send out signals along the vagus nerve to the heart. Vagal input decreases the rate with which the sinus node fires and, more importantly, *slows conduction through the AV node.*

These carotid baroreceptors are not particularly shrewd, and they can be fooled into thinking that the blood pressure is rising by gentle pressure applied *externally* to the carotid artery. (For that matter, anything that raises the blood pressure, such as a Valsalva maneuver or squatting, will stimulate vagal input to the heart, but carotid massage is the simplest and most widely used maneuver.) Since, in the majority of cases, the underlying mechanism of PSVT is a reentrant circuit involving the AV node, carotid massage may

- Interrupt the reentrant circuit and thereby terminate the arrhythmia

- At the very least, slow the arrhythmia so that the presence or absence of P waves can be more easily determined and the arrhythmia diagnosed.

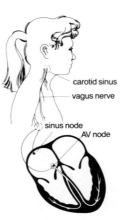

The carotid sinus contains baroreceptors that influence vagal input to the heart, primarily affecting the sinus node and AV node.

How To Do Carotid Massage

Carotid massage must be done with great care.

1. Auscultate for carotid bruits. You do *not* want to cut off the last remaining trickle of blood to the brain nor dislodge an atherosclerotic plaque. If there is evidence of significant carotid disease, do *not* perform carotid massage.

2. With the patient lying flat, extend the neck and rotate the head slightly away from you.

3. Palpate the carotid artery at the angle of the jaw and apply gentle pressure for 10 to 15 seconds.

4. *Never* compress both carotid arteries simultaneously!

5. Try the right carotid first, because the rate of success is somewhat better on this side. If it fails, however, go ahead and try the left carotid next.

6. Have a rhythm strip running during the entire procedure, so that you can see what is happening. Always have equipment for resuscitation available; in rare instances, carotid massage may induce sinus arrest.

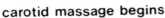

carotid massage begins

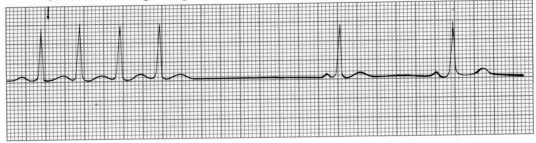

An episode of paroxysmal supraventricular tachycardia is broken almost at once by carotid massage. The new rhythm is sinus at a rate of 50 beats per minute.

Atrial Flutter

Atrial flutter is less common than PSVT. It can occur in normal hearts or, more often, in patients with underlying cardiac pathology. It, too, is absolutely regular. P waves appear at a rate of 250 to 350 beats per minute.

Atrial depolarization occurs at such a rapid rate that discrete P waves separated by a flat baseline are not seen. Instead, the baseline continually rises and falls, producing so-called *flutter waves*. In some leads, usually leads II and III, these may be quite prominent and may create what has been termed a *sawtooth pattern*.

The AV node cannot handle the extraordinary number of atrial impulses bombarding it—it simply doesn't have time to repolarize in time for each ensuing wave—and so not all of the atrial impulses pass through the AV node to generate QRS complexes. Some just bump into a refractory node and that is as far as they get. This phenomenon is called *AV block*. A 2 : 1 block is most common. This means that for every two visible flutter waves, one passes through the AV node to generate a QRS complex, and one does not. Blocks of 3 : 1 and 4 : 1 are also frequently seen. Carotid massage may increase the degree of block (*e.g.*, changing a 2 : 1 block to a 4 : 1 block), making it easier to identify the sawtooth pattern.

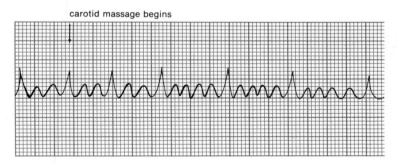

carotid massage begins

Atrial flutter. Carotid massage increases the block from 2 : 1 to 4 : 1.

Atrial Fibrillation

In *atrial fibrillation*, atrial activity is completely chaotic and the AV node may be bombarded with more than 500 impulses per minute! Whereas in atrial flutter a single constant reentrant circuit is responsible for the regular sawtooth pattern on the EKG, in atrial fibrillation the reentrant circuit is always changing in a totally unpredictable fashion. No true P waves can be seen. Instead, the baseline appears flat or undulates slightly. The AV node, faced with this extraordinary blitz of atrial impulses, allows only occasional impulses to pass through at variable intervals, generating an *irregularly irregular* ventricular rate, usually between 120 and 180 beats per minute. However, slower or faster ventricular responses (see *A* and *B* below) can often be seen.

This irregularly irregular appearance of QRS complexes in the absence of discrete P waves is the key to identifying atrial fibrillation. The wavelike forms that may often be seen on close inspection of the undulating baseline are called *fibrillation waves.*

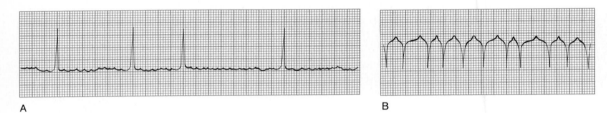

A   B

(*A*) Atrial fibrillation with a slow, irregular ventricular rate. (*B*) Another example of atrial fibrillation. In the absence of a clearly fibrillating baseline, the only clue that this rhythm is atrial fibrillation is the irregularly irregular appearance of the QRS complexes.

Carotid massage may slow the ventricular rate in atrial fibrillation, but it is rarely used in this setting because the diagnosis is usually obvious.

Atrial fibrillation is much more common than atrial flutter. Underlying cardiac pathology is often present, especially mitral valve disease or coronary artery disease, but hyperthyroidism, pulmonary emboli, and pericarditis must always be considered in the differential diagnosis.

Multifocal Atrial Tachycardia

Multifocal atrial tachycardia (MAT) is an irregular rhythm occurring at a rate of 100 to 200 beats per minute. It probably results from the random firing of several different atrial foci. Sometimes the rate is less than 100 beats per minute, in which case the arrhythmia is often called a *wandering atrial pacemaker.*

MAT is very common in patients with severe lung disease, and it rarely requires treatment. Carotid massage has *no* effect on MAT. A wandering atrial pacemaker can be seen in normal, healthy hearts.

MAT can be distinguished from atrial fibrillation by the easily identifiable P waves occurring before each QRS complex. The P waves, originating from multiple sites in the atria, will vary in shape, and the interval between the different P waves and the QRS complexes will vary as well. In order to make the diagnosis of MAT, you need to identify at least three different P wave morphologies.

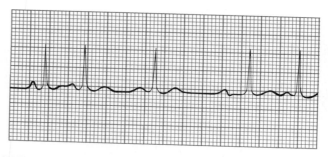

Multifocal tachycardia (MAT). Note that (1) the P waves vary dramatically in shape; (2) the PR intervals also vary; and (3) the ventricular rate is irregular.

Paroxysmal Atrial Tachycardia

The last of our five ectopic supraventricular arrhythmias, paroxysmal atrial tachycardia (PAT), is a regular rhythm with a rate of 100 to 200 beats per minute. It can result from either the enhanced automaticity of an ectopic atrial focus, or from a reentrant circuit within the atria. The automatic type typically displays a warm-up period when it starts, during which the rhythm appears somewhat irregular, and a similar cool-down period when it terminates. The less common reentrant form starts abruptly with an atrial premature beat.

PAT is most commonly seen in otherwise normal hearts. The most common underlying cause is digitalis toxicity.

How can you tell PAT from PSVT? Many times you can't. However, if you see a warm-up or cool-down period on the EKG, the rhythm is likely to be PAT. In addition, carotid massage can be very helpful: Carotid massage will slow or terminate PSVT, whereas it has virtually no effect on PAT (there may be some mild slowing).

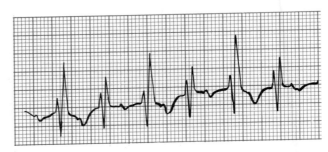

PAT. P waves are not always visible, but here they can be seen fairly easily. You may also notice the varying distance between the P waves and the ensuing QRS complexes; this reflects a varying conduction delay between the atria and ventricles that often accompanies PAT (but we are getting way ahead of ourselves; conduction delays will be discussed in Chapter 4).

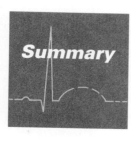

Supraventricular Arrhythmias

	Characteristics	*EKG*
PSVT	Regular Rate: 150 bpm–250 bpm Carotid massage: slows or terminates	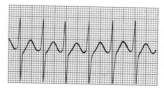
Flutter	Regular, sawtooth 2 : 1, 3 : 1, 4 : 1, etc., block Atrial rate: 250 bpm–350 bpm Ventricular rate: one half, one third, one quarter, etc., of atrial rate Carotid massage: increases block	carotid massage begins 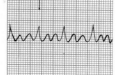
Fibrillation	Irregular Undulating baseline Atrial rate: 350 bpm–500 bpm Ventricular rate: variable Carotid massage: may slow ventricular rate	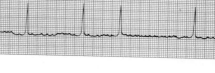
MAT	Irregular Rate: 100 bpm–200 bpm; sometimes less than 100 bpm Carotid massage: no effect	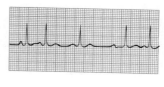
PAT	Regular Rate: 100 bpm–200 bpm Characteristic warm-up period in the automatic form Carotid massage: no effect, or only mild slowing	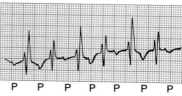 P P P P P P P

⊞ Ectopic Ventricular Arrhythmias

Ventricular arrhythmias are rhythm disturbances arising below the AV node.

Premature Ventricular Contractions

Premature ventricular contractions, or PVCs, are certainly the most common of the ventricular arrhythmias. The QRS complex of a PVC appears wide and bizarre because ventricular depolarization does not follow the normal conduction pathways. However, the QRS complex may not appear wide in all leads, so scan the entire 12-lead EKG before making your diagnosis. A retrograde P wave may sometimes be seen, but it is more common to see no P wave at all. A PVC is followed by a prolonged pause before the next beat appears.

Isolated PVCs are common in normal hearts and rarely require treatment. An isolated PVC in the setting of an acute myocardial infarction, however, is more ominous, because it can trigger ventricular tachycardia or ventricular fibrillation, both of which are life-threatening arrhythmias.

PVCs may occur randomly or may alternate with normal sinus beats in a regular pattern. If the ratio is one normal sinus beat to one PVC, the rhythm is called *bigeminy. Trigeminy* refers to two normal sinus beats for every one PVC, and so on.

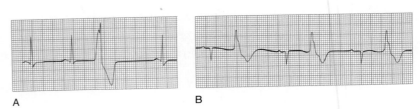

A   B

(*A*) A premature ventricular contraction. (*B*) Bigeminy. PVCs and sinus beats alternate in a 1 : 1 fashion.

When should you worry about PVCs? This is a subject of much debate, and the debate is far from over. Certain situations have been identified in which PVCs appear to pose an increased risk of triggering ventricular tachycardia, ventricular fibrillation, and death. These situations are summarized in *the rules of malignancy:*

1. Frequent PVCs

2. Runs of consecutive PVCs, especially three or more in a row

3. Multiform PVCs, in which the PVCs vary in their site of origin and hence in their appearance

4. PVCs falling on the T wave of the previous beat, called the "R on T" phenomenon. The T wave is a vulnerable period in the cardiac cycle, and a PVC falling there appears to be more likely to set off ventricular tachycardia.

5. Any PVC occurring in the setting of an acute myocardial infarction.

Although PVCs meeting one or several of these criteria are associated with an increased risk of developing a life-threatening arrhythmia, there is no evidence that suppressing these PVCs with antiarrhythmic medication reduces mortality in any setting.

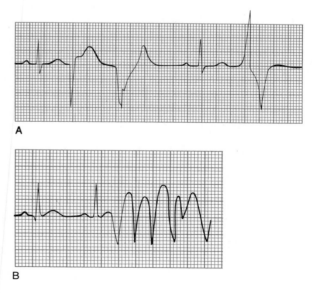

(*A*) Beats 1 and 4 are sinus in origin. The other three beats are PVCs. The PVCs differ from each other in shape (multiform), and two occur in a row. (*B*) A PVC falls on the T wave of the second sinus beat, initiating a run of ventricular tachycardia.

Ventricular Tachycardia

A run of three or more consecutive PVCs is called *ventricular tachycardia* (VT). The rate is usually between 120 and 200 beats per minute and, unlike PSVT, may be slightly irregular (although it may take a very fine eye to see this). Sustained VT is an emergency, presaging cardiac arrest and requiring immediate treatment.

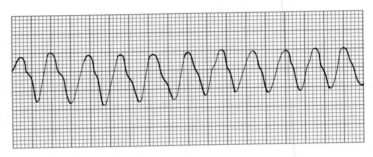

Ventricular tachycardia. The rate is about 200 beats per minute.

Ventricular Fibrillation

Ventricular fibrillation is a preterminal event. It is seen almost solely in dying hearts. It is the most frequently encountered arrhythmia in adults who experience sudden death. The EKG tracing jerks about spasmodically (coarse ventricular fibrillation) or undulates gently (fine ventricular fibrillation). There are no true QRS complexes.

In ventricular fibrillation the heart generates no cardiac output, and cardiopulmonary resuscitation and electrical defibrillation must be performed at once.

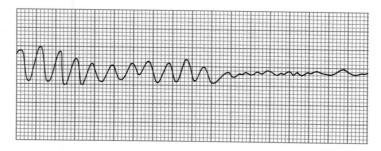

Ventricular tachycardia degenerates into ventricular fibrillation.

High-Tech Digression: The Signal-Averaged EKG

As discussed at the beginning of this section, certain types of PVCs are associated with an increased risk of developing ventricular tachycardia and ventricular fibrillation. In a further effort to identify patients who are at risk of developing sustained ventricular arrythmias, and who therefore are at risk of sudden death, electrophysiologists have been studying a technique called **signal-averaged electrocardiography** (SAECG).

We have learned that patients who develop sustained VT have a region of slower or delayed conduction in their ventricular myocardium (as expected, for this is one of the requirements for the development of a reentrant loop). This region of delayed conduction is very small and does not leave a detectable mark on the QRS complexes recorded on standard EKGs. The SAECG records numerous QRS complexes and filters out the background noise so that the tiny voltages produced by the regions of delayed conduction can be detected in the terminal portion of the QRS complexes. These abnormal voltages are called *late potentials*, and their presence has been correlated with the risk of developing life-threatening ventricular arrhythmias.

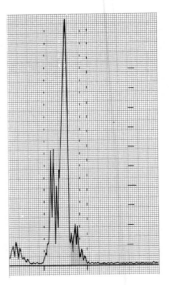

An example of SAECG. Note that the QRS complex has been tremendously enlarged. The late potential is the shaded portion at the end of the QRS complex. This tracing belongs to a patient with easily induced ventricular tachycardia.

Accelerated Idioventricular Rhythm

Accelerated idioventricular rhythm is a benign rhythm that is sometimes seen during an acute infarction. It is a regular rhythm occurring at 50 to 100 beats per minute and probably represents a ventricular escape focus that has accelerated sufficiently to drive the heart. It is rarely sustained, does not progress to ventricular fibrillation, and rarely requires treatment.

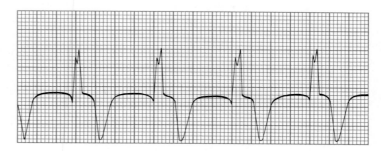

Accelerated idioventricular rhythm. There are no P waves, the QRS complexes are wide, and the rate is about 75 beats per minute.

Torsades de Pointes

Torsades de pointes, meaning "twisting of the points," is more than just the most lyrical name in cardiology. It is a unique form of VT that is usually seen in patients with prolonged QT intervals.

The QT interval, you will recall, encompasses the time from the beginning of ventricular depolarization to the end of ventricular repolarization. It normally comprises about 40% of the complete cardiac cycle.

A prolonged QT interval can be congenital in origin, or it can result from various electrolyte disturbances (notably hypocalcemia, hypomagnesemia and hypokalemia) or during an acute myocardial infarction. Numerous pharmacologic agents can also prolong the QT interval: these include quinidine and other antiarrhythmic drugs, tricyclic antidepressants, the phenothiazines, and the newer nonsedating antihistamines when taken concurrently with certain antibiotics, particularly erythromycin.

A prolonged QT interval is generally due to prolonged ventricular repolarization (that is, the T wave is lengthened). A PVC falling during the elongated T wave can initiate torsades de pointes.

Torsades de pointes looks just like ordinary, run-of-the-mill VT, except that the QRS complexes spiral around the baseline, changing their axis and amplitude. It is important to distinguish torsades de pointes from standard VT because they are treated very differently.

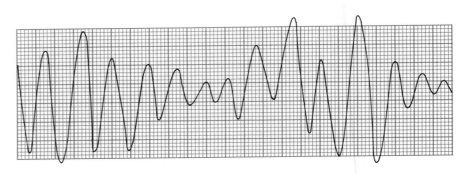

Torsades de pointes. The QRS complexes seem to spin around the baseline, changing their axis and amplitude.

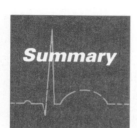

Ventricular Arrhythmias

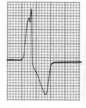 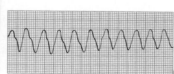 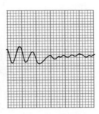

PVC   Ventricular tachycardia   Ventricular fibrillation

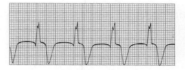 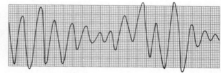

Accelerated idioventricular rhythm   Torsades de pointes

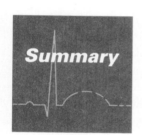

Rules of Malignancy for PVCs

Frequent PVCs

Consecutive PVCs

Multiform PVCs

R on T phenomenon

Any PVC occurring during an acute myocardial infarction (or in any patient with underlying heart disease)

⊞ *Supraventricular Versus Ventricular Arrhythmias*

The distinction between supraventricular arrhythmias and ventricular arrhythmias is extremely important, because the latter generally carry a far more ominous prognosis, and the therapy is very different. In most cases, the distinction is simple: supraventricular arrhythmias are associated with a narrow QRS complex; ventricular arrhythmias with a wide QRS complex.

There is one circumstance, however, in which supraventricular beats can produce wide QRS complexes and make the distinction considerably more difficult. This occurs when a supraventricular beat is conducted aberrantly through the ventricles, producing a wide, bizarre-looking QRS complex that is indistinguishable from a PVC. Here's how it happens.

Aberrancy

Sometimes an atrial premature beat occurs so early in the next cycle that the ventricles have not had a chance to fully repolarize in preparation for the next electrical impulse. The right bundle branch, in particular, can be particularly sluggish in this regard, and when the premature atrial impulse reaches the ventricles, the right bundle branch is still refractory. The electrical impulse is therefore prevented from passing down the right bundle branch but is able to pass quite freely down the left bundle branch (figure **A,** next page). Those areas of the ventricular myocardium ordinarily supplied by the right bundle branch must receive their electrical activation from elsewhere, namely from those areas already depolarized by the left bundle branch (figure **B,** next page). The complete process of ventricular depolarization therefore takes an unusually long time, the vector of current flow is distorted, and the result is a wide, bizarre QRS complex that looks, for all the world, like a PVC (figure **C,** next page).

(*A*) A premature atrial impulse catches the right bundle branch unprepared. Conduction down the right bundle is blocked but proceeds smoothly down the left bundle. (*B*) Right ventricular depolarization occurs only when the electrical forces can make their way over from the left ventricle—a slow, tedious process. This mode of transmission is very inefficient and results in a wide, bizarre QRS complex. (*C*) The third P wave is a premature atrial contraction. It is conducted aberrantly through the ventricles, generating a wide, bizarre QRS complex.

A wide QRS complex can therefore signify one of two things:

- A beat originating within the ventricles, or

- A supraventricular beat conducted aberrantly.

How do you tell the two apart? In the case of a single premature atrial contraction, it's usually easy, because there is a P wave preceding the wide QRS complex. Look especially closely at the T wave of the preceding beat to see if a premature P wave is hidden within it. On the other hand, and rather obviously, there is no P wave preceding a PVC.

However, when there are several consecutive beats occurring in rapid succession, or a lengthy, sustained arrhythmia, the distinction can be much more difficult. PSVT and VT have about the same rates. Thus, the tracing below is consistent with either VT or PSVT conducted aberrantly.

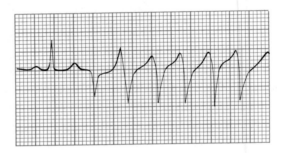

Normal sinus rhythm degenerates into a new rhythm, but is it ventricular tachycardia or supraventricular tachycardia conducted aberrantly? Don't feel bad if you can't tell. From this strip alone, as you will see, it is impossible to know for sure.

As you can see from the preceding rhythm strip, it is sometimes impossible to tell these two entities apart. There are, however, several clinical and electrocardiographic clues that can be helpful.

Clinical Clues

1. Carotid massage may terminate PSVT, whereas it has no effect on VT.

2. More than 75% of cases of VT are accompanied by *AV dissociation*. In AV dissociation, the atria and ventricles beat independently of each other. There is a ventricular pacemaker driving the ventricles and producing ventricular tachycardia on the EKG, and an independent sinus (or atrial or nodal) pacemaker driving the atria (atrial depolarization is usually hidden on the EKG by the much more prominent VT). The AV node is kept constantly refractory by the ceaseless bombardment of impulses from above and below, and therefore no impulse can cross the AV node in either direction. If, as will occur from time to time, the ventricles contract just before the atria, the atria will find themselves contracting against closed mitral and tricuspid valves. This results in a sudden back-flooding of blood into the jugular veins, producing the classic *cannon a waves* of AV dissociation. Cannon a waves are not seen in PSVT.

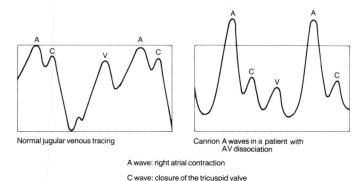

Normal jugular venous tracing   Cannon A waves in a patient with
                                                        AV dissociation

A wave: right atrial contraction

C wave: closure of the tricuspid valve

V wave: passive filling of the right atrium during diastole

Electrocardiographic Clues

1. AV dissociation can sometimes be seen on the EKG. P waves and QRS complexes march along the rhythm strip completely independently of each other. In PSVT, if P waves are seen, they bear a 1 : 1 relation to the QRS complexes. And remember, these P waves will be retrograde P waves, with a positive deflection in lead AVR and a negative deflection in lead II.

2. PSVT is regular, whereas some irregularity may be seen with VT.

3. *Fusion beats* may be seen in VT only. A fusion beat (or capture beat) occurs when an atrial impulse manages to slip through the AV node at the same time that an impulse of ventricular origin is spreading across the ventricular myocardium. The two impulses jointly depolarize the ventricles, producing a QRS complex that is morphologically part supraventricular and part ventricular.

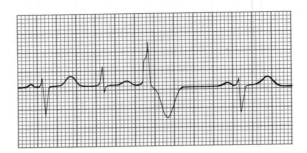

The second beat is a fusion beat, a composite of an atrial (sinus) beat (beats 1 and 4) and a PVC beat (beat 3).

4. In PSVT with aberrancy, the initial deflection of the QRS complex is usually in the same direction as that of the normal QRS complex. In VT, the initial deflection is often in the opposite direction.

None of these criteria is infallible, and sometimes it remains impossible to identify a tachyarrhythmia as ventricular or supraventricular in origin. In patients with recurrent tachycardias whose origin (and, hence, treatment) remains obscure, *His bundle electrocardiography* can be tried.

This technique is performed in the cardiac electrophysiology laboratory. A tiny catheter is placed near the region of the His bundle, and the tiny His bundle electrical potentials are recorded. If a His potential precedes every QRS complex, than a supraventricular origin is likely. If there is no relation between the His potentials and the QRS complexes, a ventricular origin is probable.

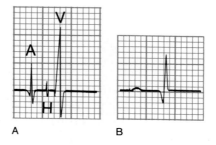

A   B

(*A*) A His bundle recording and (*B*) the corresponding EKG. In *A*, the small spike *(H)* between the spikes representing atrial and ventricular activation reflects activation of the bundle of His.

The Ashman Phenomenon

We aren't quite ready to leave the subject of aberrancy. The Ashman phenomenon is another example of aberrant conduction of a supraventricular beat. It is commonly seen in patients with atrial fibrillation.

The Ashman phenomenon describes a wide, aberrantly conducted supraventricular beat occurring *after a QRS complex that is preceded by a long pause.*

This is why it happens. The bundle branches reset their rate of repolarization according to the length of the preceding beat. If the preceding beat occurred a relatively long time ago, then the bundles repolarize somewhat leisurely. If, before repolarization is complete, another supraventricular impulse should pass through the AV node, conduction will be blocked along the normal pathways and a wide, bizarre QRS complex will be inscribed.

Atrial fibrillation, with its variable conduction producing long and short pauses between QRS complexes, is the perfect setting for this to occur.

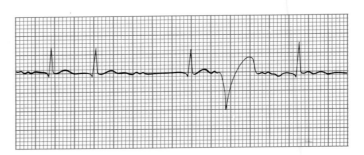

The Ashman phenomenon. The fourth beat looks like a PVC, but it could also be an aberrantly conducted supraventricular beat. Note the underlying atrial fibrillation, the short interval before the second beat, and the long interval before the third beat—all in all, a perfect substrate for the Ashman phenomenon.

Fortunately, most supraventricular arrhythmias are associated with narrow QRS complexes; aberrancy, while not uncommon, is at least the exception, not the rule. The point to take home is this: a narrow QRS complex virtually always implies a supraventricular origin, whereas a wide QRS complex usually implies a ventricular origin but may reflect aberrant conduction of a supraventricular beat.

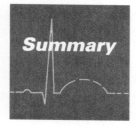

Summary

Ventricular Tachycardia (VT) Versus Paroxysmal Supraventricular Tachycardia (PSVT) With Aberrancy

	VT	*PSVT*
Clinical Clues		
Carotid massage	No response	May terminate
Cannon a waves	May be present	Not seen
EKG Clues		
AV dissociation	May be seen	Not seen
Regularity	Slightly irregular	Very regular
Fusion beats	May be seen	Not seen
Initial QRS deflection	May differ from normal QRS complex	Same as normal QRS complex

⊞ *Programmed Electrical Stimulation*

Programmed electrical stimulation (abbreviated EPS for Electrophysiologic Studies) has added a new dimension to the treatment of arrhythmias. Before the introduction of EPS, a patient with an arrhythmia requiring treatment was given a drug empirically, and after several days, when therapeutic levels had been achieved, a 24-hour Holter monitor would be used to see whether the frequency of the arrhythmia had been reduced. This hit-or-miss approach was time consuming, and exposed patients to the potential side effects of drugs that might well prove to be without benefit.

EPS is certainly not necessary for all patients with arrhythmias, and the Holter monitor remains the staple of arrhythmia diagnosis and treatment. EPS is expensive and invasive, but for certain patients it has great value, greatly refining the process of choosing the right drug for patients who need rapid and effective therapy.

The patient is taken to the electrophysiology laboratory where the particular arrhythmia is induced with intracardiac electrodes. Drugs are then infused intravenously to see whether they can suppress the inducibility of the arrhythmia. Successful suppression in the laboratory when the medication is subsequently given orally is highly correlated with successful outpatient therapy.

EPS has been used most successfully in patients who have recurrent VT or who have experienced a previous episode of sudden death requiring cardiopulmonary resuscitation.

EPS has also been used to guide surgical cures of patients with recurrent VT. Many patients with recurrent VT have a ventricular aneurysm or myocardial scar that is the source of their arrhythmia. In the operating room, the arrhythmia is induced, and the site at which depolarization begins—the origin of the arrhythmia—is mapped out. The offending area is then either resected or encircled with a deep incision.

More recently, mapping techniques have become extremely precise, and catheter ablation often mitigates the need for a more extensive surgical procedure. With this technique, it is possible to intentionally damage (*ablate*) a portion of the reentrant pathway that is the origin of the rhythm disturbance by applying electrical energy (most commonly of radio frequency) to where the catheter tip is in contact with the myocardium. The 2 or 3 mm scar that is produced usually results in a permanent cure, and the patient will not even require medication.

Here is an opportunity to review the arrhythmias we have been discussing. If you want to reexamine the basic characteristics of each arrhythmia before trying these examples, go back to the sections on arrhythmias of sinus origin, supraventricular arrhythmias, and ventricular arrhythmias. For each tracing, use the four-step method discussed previously. Always ask the following questions:

1. Are P waves present?

2. Are the QRS complexes narrow or wide?

3. What is the relationship between the P waves and the QRS complexes?

4. Is the rhythm regular or irregular?

The answers are given below.

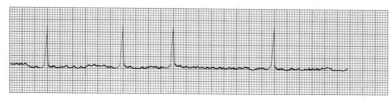

A

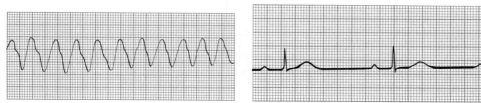

B   C

(A) Atrial fibrillation. (B) Ventricular tachycardia. (C) Sinus bradycardia. (D) Ventricular fibrillation. (E) Paroxysmal supra-ventricular tachycardia.

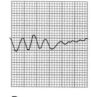

D   E

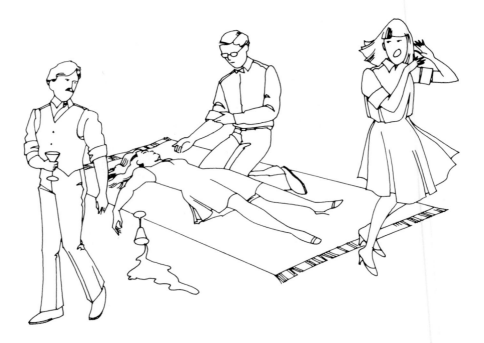

Case 3

Lola deB., predictably, is the life of the party. Never missing a turn on the dance floor nor a round at the bar, she becomes increasingly intoxicated as the evening progresses. Her husband, a young business executive, forces her to drink some coffee to sober her up before they leave. As he is wandering around in search of their coats, he hears a scream and rushes back to find her collapsed on the floor. Everyone is in a panic and all eyes turn to you, word having gotten around that you have recently been reading a well-known and highly regarded EKG book. The terror in the room is palpable, but you grin modestly, toss down a final swig of mineral water, and stride confidently to the patient saying as you go, ''Don't worry. I can handle it.''

Can you? What has happened to Lola, and just what *are* you going to do about it?

Of course a whole host of things could have happened to Lola (they usually do), but you know that the combination of alcohol, coffee and the excitement of the party can induce a *paroxysmal supraventricular tachycardia* (PSVT) in anyone, no matter how healthy they are and no matter how normal their heart. It is likely that this supraventricular rhythm disturbance has caused her to faint.

You bend down over her, assure yourself that she is breathing, and feel her pulse. It is rapid and regular with a rate of about 200 beats per minute. Since she is young and very unlikely to have significant carotid artery disease, you go right ahead and perform carotid massage, and within about 10 seconds you feel her pulse shift gears and return to normal. Her eyes blink open and the room erupts in cheers. Your guess was correct.

As you are carried out of the room on everyone's shoulders, don't forget to remind them which book you were reading that taught you all this good stuff.

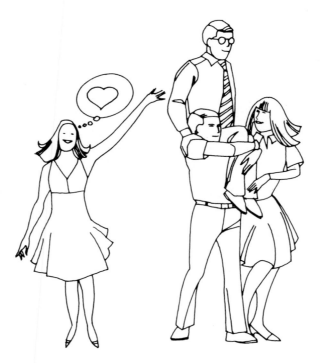

This case is so classic that no further evaluation is needed once Lola has been revived. However, many cardiologists would order a subsequent Holter monitor just to have the assurance that there is no underlying subclinical rhythm disturbance that might bear watching or even treating. In general, it will suffice to educate Lola about the merits of sobriety, or at least a more prudent approach to her evening entertainment.

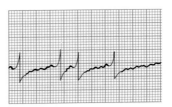

Case 4

George M., older than time, comes to see you late one Friday afternoon (he always comes late on Friday afternoons, probably because he knows you like to get an early start on the weekend and his late arrival disturbs your usual calm, professional demeanor). This time he tells you that he fainted the day before and now is feeling a bit light-headed. He also has a strange fluttering sensation in his chest. George is always complaining of something, and you have yet to find anything the matter with him in the many years you have known him, but just to be careful you obtain an EKG.

You quickly recognize the arrhythmia and are reaching for your stethoscope when George's eyes roll back in his head and he drops unconscious to the floor. Fortunately, the EKG is still running, and you see

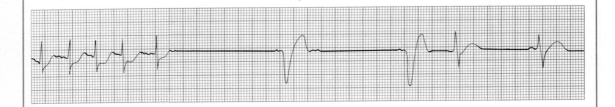

You drop down to his side, ready, if need be, to begin cardiopulmonary resuscitation, when his eyes pop open and he mutters something under his breath. The EKG now shows

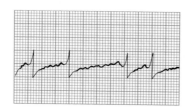

You may not know what's going on, but at least you can identify the three tracings. Right?

The first and third tracings are the same, showing classic atrial fibrillation. The baseline is undulating, without clear-cut P waves, and the QRS complexes appear irregularly. The second tracing is more interesting. It shows the atrial fibrillation terminating abruptly and then a long pause. (It was during such a pause that George dropped to the floor, a result of brain hypoxia caused by no cardiac output.) The beats that you see next are ventricular escape beats. The QRS complexes are wide and bizarre, there are no P waves, and the rate is about 33 beats per minute, exactly what you would expect of a ventricular escape rhythm. The final thing you see on the strip is the sinus node at last kicking in, albeit at a slow rate of 50 beats per minute.

George has *sick sinus syndrome,* also called the *brady-tachy syndrome.* It is typified by alternating episodes of supraventricular tachycardia and bradycardia. Often, when the supraventricular arrhythmia terminates, there is a long pause (greater than 4 seconds) before the sinus node fires again (hence the term, sick sinus). Fortunately for George, a few ventricular escape beats came to a timely rescue.

Sick sinus syndrome usually reflects significant underlying disease of the conduction system of the sort that we will be studying in the next chapter. It is one of the leading reasons for pacemaker insertion.

George M. revives in your office, and insists on going home. Fortunately, wiser heads prevail and he is taken by ambulance to the hospital. A short stay in the Cardiac Care Unit confirms that he has not had a heart attack, but his heart monitor shows numerous episodes of prolonged bradycardia alternating with various supraventricular arrhythmias. It is decided that George should have a pacemaker placed, and he reluctantly agrees. The pacemaker provides a safety net, giving George's heart an electrical "kick" everytime his own electrical mechanism fails him. George is discharged, and no further episodes of symptomatic bradycardia occur.

The Only EKG Book You'll Ever Need, second edition, by Malcolm S. Thaler.
JB Lippincott Company, Philadelphia © 1995.

Conduction Blocks

In this chapter you will learn:

1 what a conduction block is

2 that there are several types of conduction blocks that can occur between the sinus node and the AV node, some which are of little concern, and others which can be life-threatening

3 how to recognize each of these AV blocks on the EKG

4 that conduction blocks which occur in the ventricles, called bundle branch blocks, are easily identified on the EKG

5 that sometimes conduction along only a *piece* of a bundle branch can be blocked

6 how to recognize combined AV blocks and bundle branch blocks on the EKG

7 what pacemakers are used for, and what their bursts of electrical activity look like on an EKG

8 about the case of Sally M., which will illustrate the importance of knowing when conduction disturbances are truly disturbing.

⊞ *What Is a Conduction Block?*

Any obstruction of the normal pathways of electrical conduction is called a *conduction block*.

A conduction block can occur anywhere in the conduction system of the heart. There are three types of conduction blocks, defined by their anatomic location:

1. *Sinus node block*—This is the sinus exit block that we discussed in the last chapter. In this situation, the sinus node fires normally, but the wave of depolarization is immediately blocked and is not transmitted into the atrial tissue. On the EKG it looks just like a pause in the normal cardiac cycle. We will not discuss it further.

2. *AV block*—This term refers to any conduction block between the sinus node and up to and including the AV node. It is now recognized that some AV blocks occur below the AV node, but since we didn't know this until recently, the term stands.

3. *Bundle branch block*—As the name indicates, bundle branch block refers to a conduction block in one or both of the ventricular bundle branches. Sometimes only a part of one of the bundle branches is blocked; this circumstance is called a *fascicular block*.

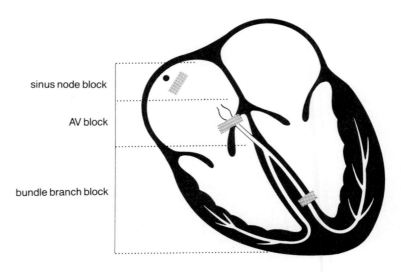

To a rough approximation, this picture shows the sites of the three major conduction blocks.

⊞ *AV Blocks*

AV blocks come in three varieties, appropriately termed *first degree, second degree,* and *third degree.* They are diagnosed by carefully examining the relationship of the P waves to the QRS complexes.

First-Degree AV Block

First-degree AV block is characterized by a prolonged delay in conduction at the AV node or His bundle (recall that the His bundle—or bundle of His, depending upon your grammatical preference—is the part of the conducting system located just below the AV node. A routine 12-lead EKG cannot distinguish between a block in the AV node and one in the His bundle). The wave of depolarization spreads normally from the sinus node through the atria, but upon reaching the AV node is held up for longer than the usual one-tenth of a second. As a result, the PR interval—the time between the start of atrial depolarization and ventricular depolarization which encompasses the delay at the AV node—is prolonged.

The diagnosis of first-degree AV block requires only that the PR interval be greater than 0.2 seconds.

In first-degree AV block, despite the delay at the AV node or His bundle, every atrial impulse does eventually make it through the AV node to activate the ventricles. Therefore, to be precise, first-degree AV block is not really a "block" at all, but rather a "delay" in conduction. Every QRS complex is preceded by a single P wave.

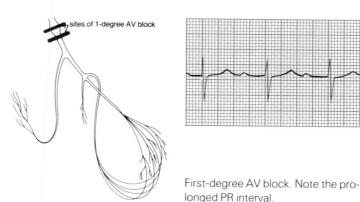

sites of 1-degree AV block

First-degree AV block. Note the prolonged PR interval.

First-degree AV block is a common finding in normal hearts, but it can also be an early sign of degenerative disease of the conduction system or a transient manifestation of myocarditis or drug toxicity. By itself, it does not require treatment.

Second-Degree AV Block

In *second-degree AV block, not* every atrial impulse is able to pass through the AV node into the ventricles. Because some P waves fail to conduct through to the ventricles, the ratio of P waves to QRS complexes is greater than 1 : 1.

Just to make things a little more interesting, there are two types of second-degree AV block: *Mobitz type I second-degree AV block,* more commonly called *Wenckebach block,* and *Mobitz type II second-degree AV block.*

Wenckebach Block

Wenckebach block is almost always due to a block within the AV node. However, the electrical effects of Wenckebach block are very different. The block, or delay, is variable, increasing with each ensuing impulse. **Each successive atrial impulse encounters a longer and longer delay in the AV node until one impulse (usually every third or fourth) fails to make it through.** What you see on the EKG is a progressive lengthening of the PR interval with each beat and then suddenly a P wave that is not followed by a QRS complex (a "dropped beat"). After this dropped beat, during which no QRS complex appears, the sequence repeats itself, over and over, and often with impressive regularity.

The example below shows a 4 : 3 Wenckebach block, in which every fourth atrial impulse fails to stimulate the ventricles, producing a ratio of four P waves to every three QRS complexes.

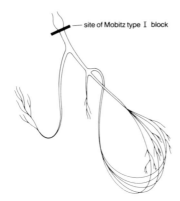

site of Mobitz type I block

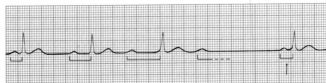

Mobitz type I second-degree AV block (Wenckebach block). The PR intervals become progressively longer until one QRS complex is dropped.

The diagnosis of Wenckebach block requires the progressive lengthening of each successive PR interval until one P wave fails to conduct through the AV node and is therefore not followed by a QRS complex.

Mobitz Type II Block

Unfortunately, this second type of second-degree AV block does not come with a more sonorous sobriquet (*i.e.* catchy nickname).

Mobitz type II block is due to a block *below* the AV node in the His bundle. It resembles Wenckebach block in that some, but not all, of the atrial impulses are transmitted to the ventricles. However, progressive lengthening of the PR interval does *not* occur. Instead, conduction is an all-or-nothing phenomenon. The EKG shows two or more normal beats with normal PR intervals and than a P wave that is not followed by a QRS complex (a dropped beat). The cycle is then repeated. The ratio of conducted beats to nonconducted beats is rarely constant, with the ratio of P waves to QRS complexes constantly varying, from 2 : 1 to 3 : 2 and so on.

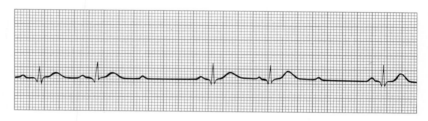

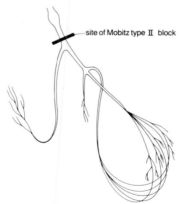

site of Mobitz type II block

Mobitz type II second-degree AV block. On the EKG, every third P wave is not followed by a QRS complex (dropped beat).

The diagnosis of Mobitz type II block requires the presence of a dropped beat without progressive lengthening of the PR interval.

Is It a Wenckebach Block or a Mobitz Type II Block?

Compare the electrocardiographic manifestations of Wenckebach block and Mobitz type II block on the EKGs below:

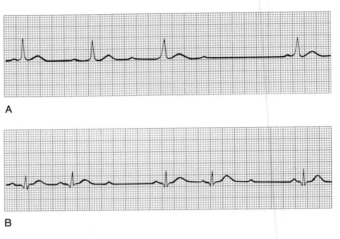

A

B

(*A*) Wenckebach block, with progressive lengthening of the PR interval.
(*B*) Mobitz type II block, in which the PR interval is constant.

Now that you are an expert, look at the EKG below. Is this an example of Wenckebach block or Mobitz type II block?

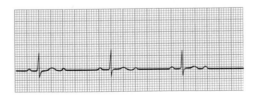

Well, it certainly is an example of second-degree heart block with a P wave to QRS complex ratio of 2 : 1, but you were pretty clever if you realized that it is impossible to tell whether it is due to Wenckebach block or Mobitz type II block. The distinction between these two types of second-degree heart block depends on whether or not there is progressive PR lengthening, but with a 2 : 1 ratio in which every other QRS complex is dropped, it is impossible to make this determination.

When circumstances permit a more accurate determination, the distinction between Wenckebach block and Mobitz type II second-degree AV block is an important one to make.

Wenckebach block is usually due to a conduction block high up in the AV node. It is typically transient and benign, and rarely progresses to a third-degree heart block (see next page) which can be dangerous and even life-threatening.

Mobitz type II block is usually due to a conduction block below the AV node, somewhere in the His bundle. Although less common than Wenckebach block, it is far more serious, often signifying serious heart disease and capable of progressing suddenly to third-degree heart block.

Whereas treatment is often not needed for Wenckebach block, Mobitz type II heart block often mandates insertion of a pacemaker.

Some technical gibberish you should probably ignore. In cases of 2 : 1 second-degree AV block, as shown on the previous page, there is a way to localize the site of the block and determine how serious the problem may be. Can you think of how to do it?

His bundle electrocardiography, as described previously, will do the job. A small electrode introduced into the region of the His bundle can identify whether the site of the block is above, within, or below the His bundle, and therefore can accurately predict the patient's prognosis, *i.e.* the likelihood of progression to third-degree heart block.

Third-Degree AV Block

Third-degree heart block is the ultimate in heart blocks. *No* atrial impulses make it through to activate the ventricles. For this reason it is often called *complete heart block*. The site of the block can be either at the AV node or lower. The ventricles respond to this dire situation by generating an escape rhythm, usually an inadequate 30 to 45 beats per minute. The atria and ventricles continue to contract, but they now do so at their own intrinsic rates, approximately 60 to 100 beats per minute for the atria, and 30 to 45 beats per minute for the ventricles. In complete heart block, the atria and ventricles have virtually nothing to do with each other, separated by the absolute barrier of the complete conduction block. We have already described this type of situation in our discussion of ventricular tachycardia: it is called *AV dissociation* and refers to any circumstance in which the atria and ventricles are being driven by independent pacemakers.

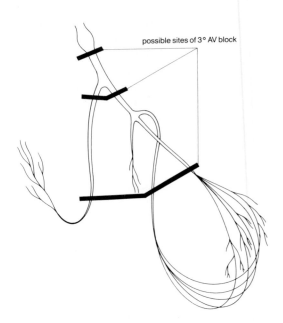

possible sites of 3° AV block

The EKG in third-degree heart block shows P waves marching across the rhythm strip at their usual rate (60 to 100 waves per minute) but bearing no relationship to the QRS complexes that appear at a much slower escape rate. The QRS complexes appear wide and bizarre, just like PVCs, because they arise not from the usual conduction pathways but from a ventricular source.

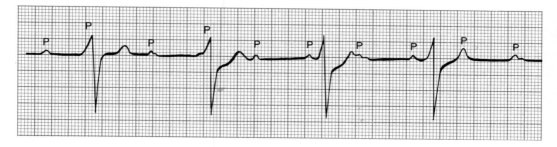

Third-degree AV block. The P waves appear at regular intervals, as do the QRS complexes, but they have nothing to do with one another. The QRS complexes are wide, implying a ventricular origin.

Although a ventricular escape rhythm may look like a slow run of PVCs (slow ventricular tachycardia), there is one important difference: PVCs are *premature*, occurring before the next expected beat, and even the slowest VT will be faster than the patient's normal rhythm. A ventricular escape beat occurs after a long pause, and is therefore never premature, and a sustained ventricular escape rhythm is always *slower* than the normal beats. PVCs, being premature intrusions, can be suppressed with little clinical consequence. A ventricular escape rhythm, however, may be lifesaving, and suppression could be fatal.

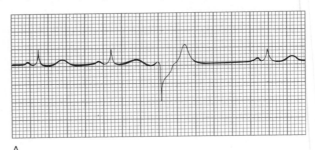

A

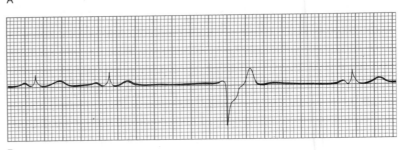

B

(*A*) The third beat is a PVC, occurring before the next anticipated normal beat.
(*B*) The third ventricular complex occurs late, after a prolonged pause. This is a ventricular escape beat.

The diagnosis of third-degree heart block requires the presence of AV dissociation in which the ventricular rate is slower than the sinus or atrial rate.

Degenerative disease of the conduction system is the leading cause of third-degree heart block. It can also complicate an acute myocardial infarction. Pacemakers are virtually always required when third-degree heart block develops. It is a true medical emergency.

Some forms of complete heart block develop prenatally (congenital heart block) and are often associated with an adequate and stable ventricular escape rhythm. Permanent pacemakers are only implanted in these children if there is clearcut developmental impairment that can be attributed to an inadequate cardiac output.

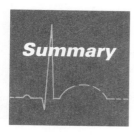

AV Block

AV block is diagnosed by examining the relationship of the P waves to the QRS complexes.

1. *First degree:* The PR interval is greater than 0.2 seconds; *all* beats are conducted through to the ventricles.

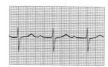

2. *Second degree:* Only *some* beats are conducted through to the ventricles.

   a. *Mobitz type I* (Wenckebach): Progressive prolongation of the PR interval until a QRS is dropped

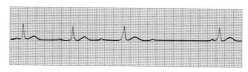

   b. *Mobitz type II:* All-or-nothing conduction, in which QRS complexes are dropped without prolongation of the PR interval

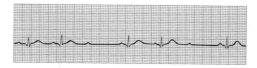

3. *Third degree:* No beats are conducted through to the ventricles. There is complete heart block with AV dissociation, in which the atria and ventricles are driven by independent pacemakers.

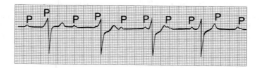

Note: Different degrees of AV block can coexist in the same patient. Thus, for example, a patient can have both first-degree and Mobitz type II heart block. Blocks also can be transient, and a patient may, for example, at one point have a second-degree block and later develop third-degree block.

⊞ *Bundle Branch Block*

The term *bundle branch block* refers to a conduction block in either the left or right bundle branches. The figure below reviews the anatomy of the ventricular bundle branches.

A Quick Review of Ventricular Depolarization

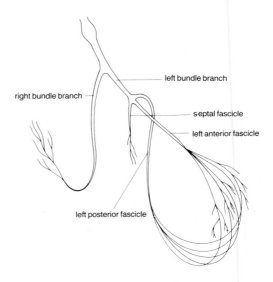

The anatomy of the ventricular bundle branches.

The normal sequence of ventricular activation should be familiar to you by now. The wave of depolarization sweeps out of the AV node and bundle of His into the bundle branch system. The right and left bundle branches deliver the current to the right and left ventricles, respectively. This is the most efficient means of dispersing the electrical current, and the resultant QRS complex, representing ventricular depolarization from start to finish, is narrow—less than 0.1 seconds in duration. Also, because the muscle mass of the left ventricle is so much larger than that of the right ventricle, left ventricular electrical forces dominate those of the right ventricle, and the resultant electrical axis is leftward, lying between 0° and +90°.

Thus, with normal ventricular depolarization, the QRS complex is narrow and the electrical axis is between 0° and 90°. **All of this changes with bundle branch block.**

Bundle branch block is diagnosed by looking at the width and configuration of the QRS complexes.

Right Bundle Branch Block

In *right bundle branch block,* conduction through the right bundle is obstructed. As a result, right ventricular depolarization is delayed; it does not begin until the left ventricle is almost fully depolarized. This causes two things to happen on the EKG:

1. The delay in right ventricular depolarization prolongs the total time for ventricular depolarization. As a result, the QRS complex widens beyond 0.12 seconds.

2. The wide QRS complex assumes a unique, virtually diagnostic shape in those leads overlying the right ventricle, V_1, and V_2. As you know, the normal QRS complex in these leads consists of a small positive R wave and a deep negative S wave, reflecting the electrical dominance of the left ventricle. With right bundle branch block, you can still see the initial R and S waves as the left ventricle depolarizes, but as the right ventricle then begins its delayed depolarization, unopposed by the now fully depolarized and electrically silent left ventricle, the electrical axis of current flow swings sharply back toward the right. This inscribes a *second* R wave, called R′, in leads V_1 and V_2. The whole complex is called RSR′, and its appearance has been likened to rabbit ears. Meanwhile, in the left lateral leads overlying the left ventricle (I, AVL, V_5, and V_6), late right ventricular depolarization causes reciprocal late deep S waves to be inscribed.

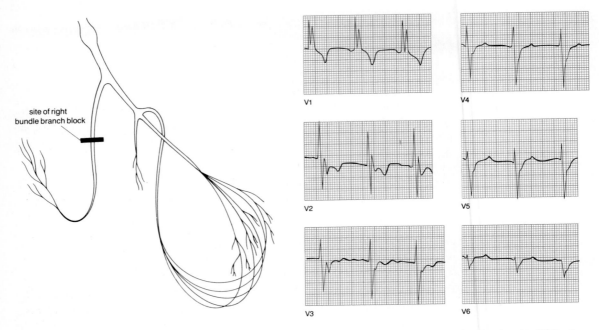

Right bundle branch block. The QRS complex in lead V_1 shows the classic wide RSR prime configuration. Note, too, the S waves in V_5 and V_6.

Left Bundle Branch Block

In *left bundle branch block*, it is *left* ventricular depolarization that is delayed. Again, there are two things to look for on the EKG:

1. The delay in left ventricular depolarization causes the QRS complex to widen beyond 0.12 seconds in duration.

2. The QRS complex in the leads overlying the left ventricle (I, AVL, V_5, and V_6) will show a characteristic change in shape. The QRS complexes in these leads already have tall R waves. Delayed left ventricular depolarization causes a marked prolongation in the rise of those tall R waves, which will either be broad on top or notched. True rabbit ears are less common than in right bundle branch block. Those leads overlying the right ventricle will show reciprocal, broad, deep S waves. The left ventricle is so dominant in left bundle branch block that left axis deviation may also be present, but this is variable.

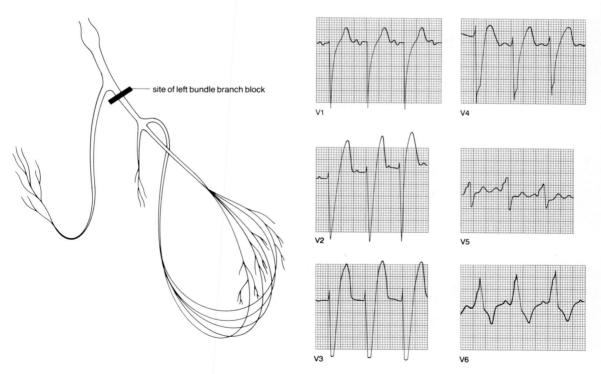

site of left bundle branch block

Left bundle branch block.

Bundle Branch Block and Repolarization

In both right and left bundle branch block, the repolarization sequence is also affected.

In right bundle branch block, the right precordial leads will show ST segment depression and T wave inversion, just like the strain pattern that occurs with ventricular hypertrophy.

Similarly, in left bundle branch block, ST segment depression and T wave inversion can be seen in the left lateral leads.

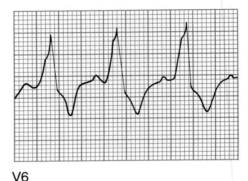

V6

ST segment depression and T wave inversion in lead V_6 in a patient with left bundle branch block.

Who Gets Bundle Branch Blocks?

Although right bundle branch block can be caused by diseases of the conducting system, it is also a fairly common phenomenon in otherwise normal hearts.

Left bundle branch block, on the other hand, rarely occurs in normal hearts and almost always reflects significant underlying cardiac disease, such as degenerative disease of the conduction system or ischemic coronary artery disease.

Critical Rate

Both right and left bundle branch block can be intermittent or fixed. In some individuals, bundle branch block only appears when a particular heart rate, called the *critical rate,* is achieved. In other words, the ventricles conduct normally at slow heart rates, but, above a certain rate, bundle branch block develops.

The development of a rate-related bundle branch block is directly related to the time it takes a particular bundle branch to repolarize and thus prepare itself for the next electrical impulse to come down the pass. If the heart rate is so rapid that a particular bundle branch cannot repolarize in time, there will be a temporary block to conduction, resulting in the classic EKG appearance of a rate related bundle branch block.

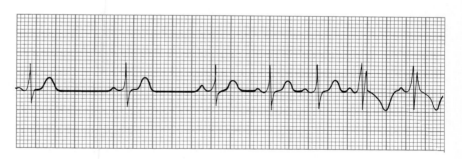

An example of critical rate (lead V₂). As the heart accelerates, the pattern of right bundle branch block appears.

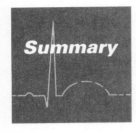

Bundle Branch Block

Bundle branch block is diagnosed by looking at the width and configuration of the QRS complexes.

Criteria for Right Bundle Branch Block

1. QRS complex widened to greater than 0.12 seconds

2. RSR' in V_1 and V_2 (rabbit ears) with ST segment depression and T wave inversion

3. Reciprocal changes in V_5, V_6, I, and AVL.

Criteria for Left Bundle Branch Block

1. QRS complex widened to greater than 0.12 seconds

2. Broad or notched R wave with prolonged upstroke in leads V_5, V_6, I, and AVL with ST segment depression and T wave inversion

3. Reciprocal changes in V_1 and V_2

4. Left axis deviation may be present.

Note: Because bundle branch block affects the size and appearance of R waves, the criteria for ventricular hypertrophy discussed in Chapter 2 cannot be used if bundle branch block is present. Specifically, right bundle branch block precludes the diagnosis of right ventricular hypertrophy, and left bundle branch block precludes the diagnosis of left ventricular hypertrophy. In addition, the diagnosis of a myocardial infarction cannot be made in the presence of left bundle branch block; we will see why in Chapter 6.

⊞ *Hemiblocks*

Here again is a picture of the ventricular conduction system. The left bundle branch is composed of three separate fascicles. These are illustrated below and include the septal fascicle, the left anterior fascicle, and the left posterior fascicle. The term *hemiblock* refers to a conduction block of just one of these fascicles. The right bundle branch does not divide into separate fascicles.

Septal blocks need not concern us here. Hemiblocks of the anterior and posterior fascicles, however, are both common and important.

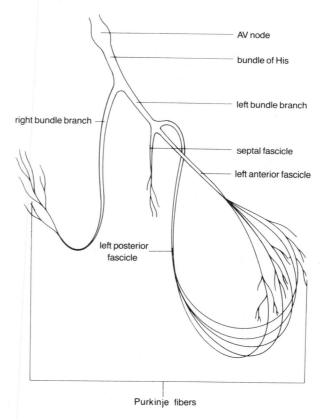

The ventricular conduction system. The right bundle branch remains intact, whereas the left bundle branch divides into three separate fascicles.

Hemiblocks Cause Axis Deviation

The major effect that hemiblocks have on the EKG is *axis deviation*. Here is why.

As shown on the previous page, the left anterior fascicle lies superiorly and laterally to the left posterior fascicle. With *left anterior hemiblock*, conduction down the left anterior fascicle is blocked. All the current therefore rushes down the left posterior fascicle to the inferior surface of the heart. Left ventricular myocardial depolarization then occurs, progressing in an inferior-to-superior and right-to-left direction.

The axis of ventricular depolarization is therefore redirected upward and slightly leftward, inscribing tall positive R waves in the left lateral leads and deep S waves inferiorly. This results in *left axis deviation* (*i.e.*, the electrical axis of ventricular depolarization is redirected between 0° and −90°).

(Do you remember how to identify left axis deviation? The simplest method is to look at the QRS complex in leads I and AVF. The QRS complex will be positive in lead I and negative in lead AVF. If you need to, refer to Chapter 2 for a quick review.)

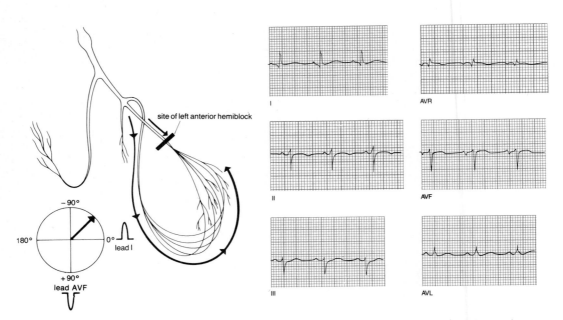

Left anterior hemiblock. Current flow down the left anterior fascicle is blocked, so all the current must pass down the posterior fascicle. The resultant axis is redirected upward and leftward (left axis deviation).

In *left posterior hemiblock,* the reverse occurs. All of the current rushes down the left anterior fascicle, and ventricular myocardial depolarization then ensues in a superior-to-inferior and left-to-right direction. The axis of depolarization is therefore directed downward and rightward, writing tall R waves inferiorly and deep S waves in the left lateral leads. The result is *right axis deviation* (*i.e.,* the electrical axis of ventricular depolarization is between +90° and 180°).

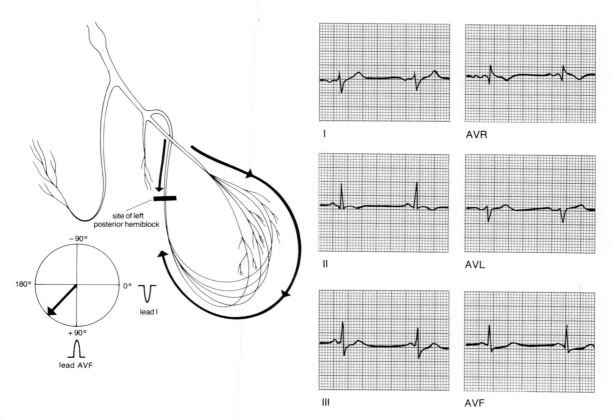

Left posterior hemiblock. Current flow down the left posterior fascicle is blocked, so all the current must pass down the right anterior fascicle. The resultant axis is redirected downward and rightward (right axis deviation).

Hemiblocks Do Not Prolong the QRS Complex

Whereas the QRS complex is widened in *complete* left and right bundle branch block, the QRS duration in both left anterior and left posterior hemiblock is normal. (Actually, there is a very minor prolongation, but not enough to widen the QRS complex appreciably.) There are also no ST segment and T wave changes.

Left anterior hemiblock is far more common than left posterior hemiblock, possibly because the anterior fascicle is longer, thinner, and has a more tenuous blood supply than the posterior fascicle. Left anterior hemiblock can be seen in both normal and diseased hearts, whereas left posterior hemiblock is virtually the exclusive province of sick hearts.

Is hemiblock present in the EKG below?

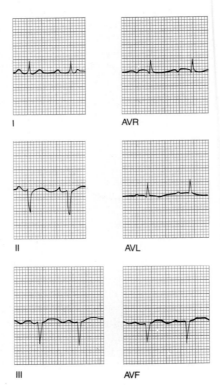

Left axis deviation indicates the presence of left anterior hemiblock.

Before settling on the diagnosis of hemiblock, it is always necessary to make sure that other causes of axis deviation, such as ventricular hypertrophy, are not present. In addition, as we shall discuss later, patients with certain clinical disorders, such as those with severe chronic lung disease, are predisposed to right axis deviation. Nevertheless, for most individuals, if the tracing is normal *except for the presence of axis deviation,* you can feel reasonably confident that hemiblock is responsible.

Criteria for Hemiblock

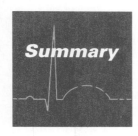
Summary

Hemiblock is diagnosed by looking for left or right axis deviation.

Left Anterior Hemiblock

1. Normal QRS duration and no ST segment or T wave changes

2. Left axis deviation

3. No other cause of left axis deviation is present.

Left Posterior Hemiblock

1. Normal QRS duration and no ST segment or T wave changes

2. Right axis deviation

3. No other cause of right axis deviation is present.

⊞ *Combining Bundle Branch Blocks and Hemiblocks*

Bundle branch blocks and hemiblocks can occur in various combinations. The term *bifascicular block* refers to the combination of either left anterior or left posterior hemiblock with right bundle branch block. In bifascicular block, only one fascicle of the left bundle branch is supplying the bulk of both ventricles. The EKG findings include a combination of features of both hemiblock and right bundle branch block.

Criteria for Bifascicular Block

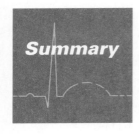

The features of right bundle branch block combined with left anterior hemiblock are as follows:

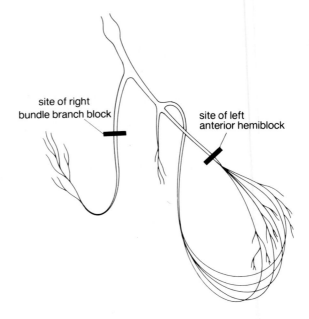

site of right
bundle branch block

site of left
anterior hemiblock

Right Bundle Branch Block

- QRS wider than 0.12 seconds

- RSR′ in V_1 and V_2.

Left Anterior Hemiblock

- Left axis deviation.

The features of right bundle branch block combined with left posterior hemiblock are as follows:

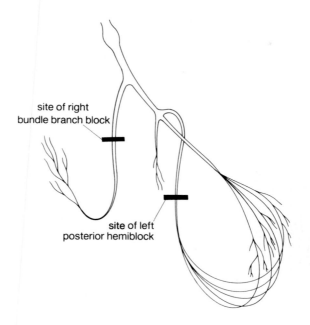

Right Bundle Branch Block

- QRS wider than 0.12 seconds
- RSR′ in V_1 and V_2.

Left Posterior Hemiblock

- Right axis deviation.

Can you identify a bifascicular block on this EKG?

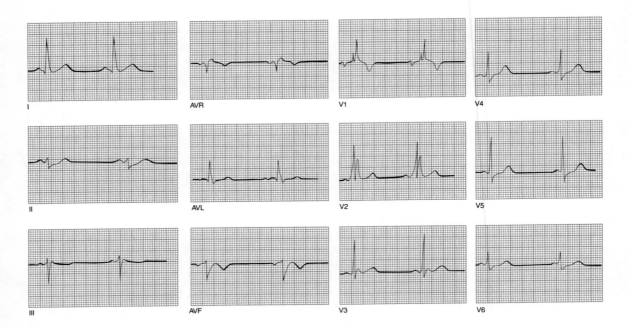

This is an example of right bundle branch block combined with left anterior hemiblock. Note the widened QRS complex and rabbit ears in leads V_1 and V_2, characteristic of right bundle branch block, and the left axis deviation in the limb leads (the QRS complex is predominantly positive in lead I and negative in lead AFV) that suggests left anterior hemiblock.

⊞ The Ultimate in Playing With Blocks: Combining AV Blocks, Bundle Branch Blocks, and Hemiblocks

Bundle branch block, hemiblocks, and bifascicular blocks can also occur in combination with AV blocks. (Are you sure you're ready for this?) Take a look at this EKG and see if you can identify the different conduction blocks that are present. An orderly approach is essential.

1. Is there any AV block?
   Look at the relationship between the P waves and QRS complexes.

2. Is there any bundle branch block?
   Look in the precordial leads for wide QRS complexes with their distinctive configurations; are there any ST segment and T wave changes?

3. Is there any hemiblock?
   Look for axis deviation.

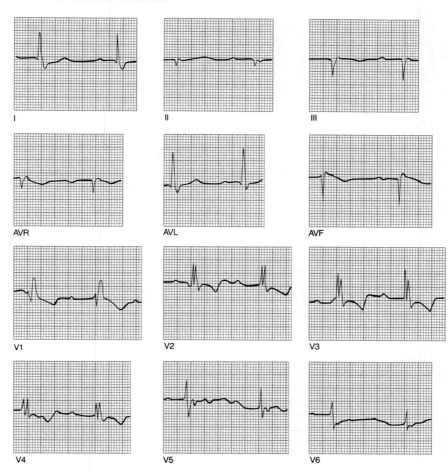

The preceding EKG shows:

1. First-degree AV block (the PR interval exceeds 0.20 seconds)

2. Right bundle branch block (there are wide QRS complexes with rabbit ears in leads V_1 through V_4)

3. Left anterior hemiblock (left axis deviation is present).

⊞ *Pacemakers*

A tremendous number of pacemakers are inserted in patients every year in the United States. There is little doubt that many of these have been inserted for questionable indications, but in the right circumstances they can be of tremendous clinical benefit. Clinical evidence strongly supports their use in patients with:

- Third-degree (complete) AV block

- A lesser degree of AV block or bradycardia (*e.g.*, sick sinus syndrome) if the patient is symptomatic

- The sudden development of various combinations of AV block and bundle branch block in patients who are in the throes of an acute myocardial infarction

- Patients with recurrent tachycardias that can be overdriven and thereby terminated by pacemaker activity.

Pacemakers are nothing more than a power source connected to electrodes. The power source is usually placed subcutaneously, and the electrodes are threaded to the right atrium or right ventricle through veins that drain to the heart. Pacemakers provide an alternate source of electrical power for a heart whose own intrinsic source of electricity (the sinus node), or whose ability to conduct electrical current, is impaired.

Pacemaker technology has accelerated dramatically in recent years. Whereas early pacemakers were capable of firing only at a single predetermined rate (*fixed rate pacemakers*) no matter what the heart itself was doing, today's pacemakers are responsive to the moment-to-moment needs of the heart. They have become completely programmable in terms of sensitivity, rate of firing, refractory period, and so on. The present generation of pacemakers can even increase the heart rate in response to motion or increased respirations for those patients who cannot increase their own heart rate appropriately during activity, either because of disease of the sinus node or the effects of medications.

The most popular pacemaker today is a *demand pacemaker*. A demand pacemaker fires only when the patient's own intrinsic heart rate falls below a threshold level. For example, a demand pacemaker set at 60 beats per minute will remain silent as long as the patient's heart rate remains above 60 beats per minute. As soon as there is a pause between beats that would translate into a rate below 60, the pacemaker will fire.

A ventricular pacemaker, in which the electrode is inserted in the wall of the right ventricle, is usually preferred unless the atrial kick is needed to maintain an adequate cardiac output. In that circumstance, an atrial pacemaker may be used. In patients with third-degree (complete) heart block who need an atrial kick, an atrial pacemaker alone is inadequate, because any atrial impulse will fail to conduct to the ventricles. For these patients, a sequential AV pacemaker can be used. Electrodes are then placed in both the right atrium and right ventricle. They are timed to fire in a sequential manner such that the atria contract first and are able to empty almost completely before the ventricles are stimulated to contract.

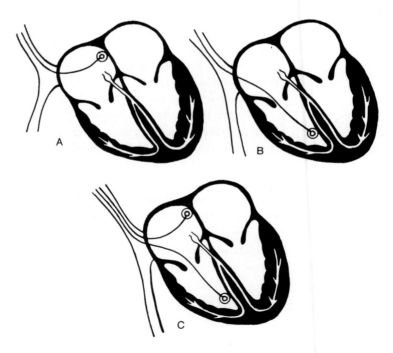

(*A*) Site of atrial pacemaker implantation. (*B*) Ventricular pacemaker. (*C*) Sequential pacemaker with atrial and ventricular leads.

When a pacemaker fires, a small spike can be seen on the EKG. With a ventricular pacemaker, the ensuing QRS complex will be wide and bizarre, just like a PVC. Because the electrodes are located in the right ventricle, the right ventricle will contract first, then the left ventricle. This generates a pattern identical to left bundle branch block, with delayed left ventricular activation. A retrograde P wave may or may not be seen.

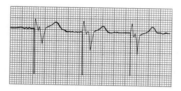

(*A*) EKG from a patient with a ventricular pacemaker.

An atrial pacemaker will generate a spike followed by a P wave and a normal QRS complex.

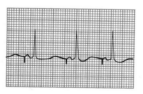

(*B*) EKG from a patient with an atrial pacemaker.

With a sequential pacemaker, two spikes will be seen, one preceding a P wave and one preceding a wide, bizarre QRS complex.

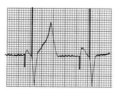

(*C*) EKG from a patient with a sequential pacemaker.

When used appropriately, pacemakers save lives. They can, however, be very dangerous even in the best of circumstances. The pacemaker spike itself always has the potential to induce a serious arrhythmia. For example, if a ventricular pacemaker should happen to fire mistakenly during the vulnerable period of ventricular repolarization (remember the R on T phenomenon?), ventricular tachycardia can be induced.

Case 5

Sally M. works at your hospital as a volunteer. One day she is instructed to take some intravenous solutions from the pharmacy in the hospital basement to the intensive care unit on the third floor. She enters the elevator with her transport cart, winking a friendly eye at the pharmacist.

You just happen to be standing at the third floor elevator, waiting impatiently for a ride down to the cafeteria. When the elevator door opens, you find Sally collapsed on the floor, motionless except for some deep gasping breaths. A quick purview of her vital signs reveals that she is stable. You grab a gurney that is conveniently parked nearby and rush her to the intensive care unit.

On the way to the unit you try talking to her. She is quite confused and disoriented, and you notice that she has been incontinent. In the ICU, this rhythm strip is obtained:

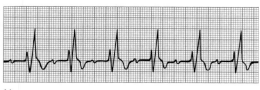

V₁

Does this rhythm strip tell you what happened to Sally on the elevator?

(continued)

In a word, no. The rhythm strip reveals a modest sinus tachycardia, first-degree AV block, and the rabbit ears of right bundle branch block. Nothing here can account for her collapse. Had you found significant bradycardia, ventricular arrhythmia, or an advanced degree of heart block, you would certainly have cause to suspect the presence of Stokes-Adams syncope, *i.e.,* a sudden faint from inadequate cardiac output. The period of disorientation following her collapse is also not typical for Stokes-Adams syncope, but is typical of the postictal state seen after a seizure.

About 15 minutes after her collapse, Sally's mental state has returned to normal and she is anxious to return to work. You are able to persuade her that a short stay in the ICU for observation would be a good idea. Continual cardiac monitoring reveals no significant arrythmias or conduction blocks, but an MRI of her head does reveal a probable meningioma. It is likely, therefore, that Sally did suffer a seizure caused by an expanding brain lesion. The meningioma is excised without complication, and several months later you see Sally happily plying her trade once again, a joyful reminder to all that performing a service for others is the surest way to achieve true satisfaction in life.

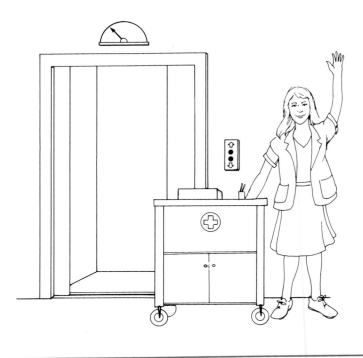

The Only EKG Book You'll Ever Need, second edition, by Malcolm S. Thaler. JB Lippincott Company, Philadelphia © 1995.

5 Preexcitation Syndromes

In this chapter you will learn:

1 what happens when electrical current is conducted to the ventricles more rapidly than usual

2 what an accessory pathway is

3 that the names Wolff-Parkinson-White and Lown-Ganong-Levine are not the names of law firms

4 why accessory pathways predispose to arrhythmias

5 about the case of Winston T., a *preexcitable* personality.

⊞ *What Is Preexcitation?*

In the last chapter we discussed what happens when conduction from the atria to the ventricles is delayed or blocked. This chapter presents the other side of the coin: what happens when the electrical current is conducted to the ventricles *more quickly than usual.*

How can such a thing happen?

With normal conduction, the major delay between the atria and the ventricles is in the AV node, where the wave of depolarization is held up for about 0.1 seconds, long enough for the atria to contract and empty their contents into the ventricles. In the *preexcitation syndromes,* there are *accessory pathways* by which the current can bypass the AV node and thus arrive at the ventricles ahead of time.

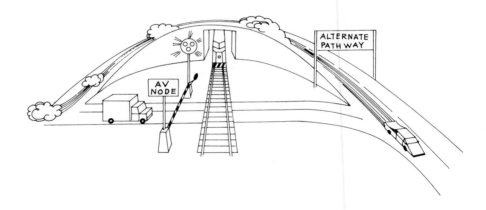

A number of different accessory pathways have been discovered. Probably fewer than 1% of individuals possess one of these pathways. There is a decided male preponderance. Accessory pathways may occur in normal healthy hearts as an isolated finding, or they may occur in conjunction with mitral valve prolapse, IHSS, and various congenital disorders.

There are two major preexcitation syndromes: *Wolff-Parkinson-White (WPW) syndrome,* and *Lown-Ganong-Levine (LGL) syndrome.* They are both easily diagnosed on the EKG. In both syndromes, the accessory conduction pathways act as short circuits, allowing the atrial wave of depolarization to by-pass the AV node and activate the ventricles prematurely.

⊞ *Wolff-Parkinson-White Syndrome*

In Wolff-Parkinson-White (WPW) syndrome, the bypass pathway has been named the **bundle of Kent.** It is a discrete aberrant conducting pathway that connects the atria and ventricles. It can be left-sided (connecting the left atrium and left ventricle) or right-sided (connecting the right atrium and right ventricle).

Premature ventricular depolarization via the bundle of Kent causes two things to happen on the EKG:

1. The PR interval, representing the time from the start of atrial depolarization to the start of ventricular depolarization, is shortened. The criterion for diagnosis is a *PR interval less than 0.12 seconds.*

2. The QRS complex is widened to more than 0.1 seconds. Unlike bundle branch block, in which the QRS complex is widened because of *delayed* ventricular activation, in WPW it is widened because of *premature* activation. The QRS complex in WPW actually represents a fusion beat: most of the ventricular myocardium is activated via the normal conduction pathways, but a small region is depolarized early via the bundle of Kent. This small region of myocardium that is depolarized early gives the QRS complex a characteristic slurred initial upstroke called a *delta wave.* A true delta wave may be seen in only a few leads, so scan the entire EKG.

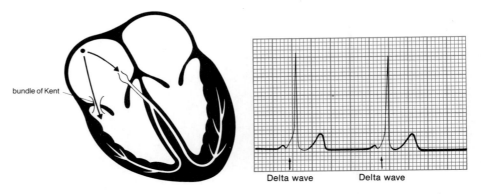

Wolff-Parkinson-White (WPW) syndrome. Current is held up by the normal delay at the AV node but races unimpeded down the bundle of Kent. The EKG shows the short PR interval and delta wave.

Lown-Ganong-Levine Syndrome

In LGL syndrome, the accessory pathway (called James fibers) is effectively *intra*-nodal. The James fibers bypass the delay within the AV node. All ventricular conduction occurs via the usual ventricular conduction pathways; unlike WPW, there is no small region of ventricular myocardium that is depolarized independently of the rest of the ventricles. Therefore, there is no delta wave, and the QRS complex is not widened. The only electrical manifestation of LGL is a shortening of the PR interval as a result of the accessory pathway bypassing the delay within the AV node.

The criteria for the diagnosis of LGL are:

The PR interval is shortened to less than 0.12 seconds

The QRS complex is not widened

There is no delta wave.

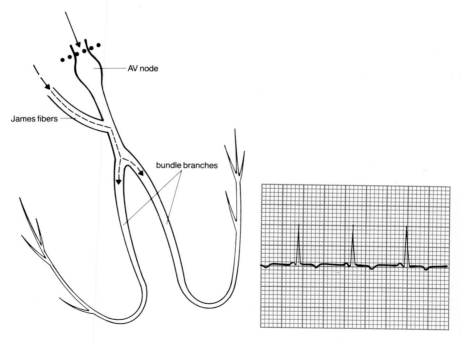

In Lown-Ganong-Levine (LGL) syndrome, the PR interval is short, but there is no delta wave.

▦ *Associated Arrhythmias*

In many individuals with WPW or LGL, preexcitation poses few, if any, clinical problems. However, it is now well established that preexcitation does predispose to various tachyarrhythmias. This predisposition has been most clearly documented in WPW, where it is estimated that 50% to 70% of individuals experience at least one supraventricular arrhythmia.

The two tachyarrhythmias most often seen in WPW are *paroxysmal supraventricular tachycardia* and *atrial fibrillation*.

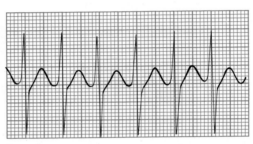

A

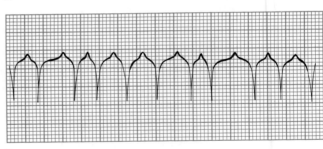

B

(*A*) Paroxysmal supraventricular tachycardia. (*B*) Atrial fibrillation.

Paroxysmal Supraventricular Tachycardia in WPW

In normal hearts, paroxysmal supraventricular tachycardia (PSVT) usually arises via a reentrant mechanism. The same is true in WPW. In fact, the presence of an accessory bundle—an alternate pathway of conduction—is the *perfect* substrate for reentry. Here is how it works.

We have already seen how, in WPW, a normal beat generates a QRS complex that is a fusion of two waves, one conducted via the bundle of Kent (the delta wave) and one via the normal route of conduction. Although the bundle of Kent usually conducts current faster than the AV node, it also tends to have a longer refractory period once it has been depolarized. What happens, then, if a normal sinus impulse is followed abruptly by a premature atrial beat? This premature beat will be conducted normally through the AV node, but the bundle of Kent may still be refractory, blocking conduction via the alternate route. The wave of depolarization will then move through the AV node and into the bundle branches and ventricular myocardium. By the time it encounters the bundle of Kent on the ventricular side, it may no longer be refractory and the current can pass back into the atria. It is then free to pass right back down through the AV node, and a self-sustaining, revolving reentrant mechanism has been established. The result is PSVT. The QRS complex is narrow because ventricular depolarization occurs via the normal bundle branches.

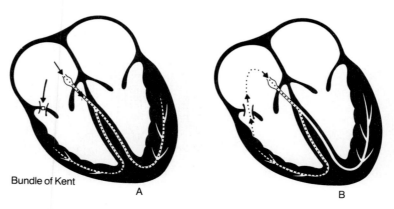

Bundle of Kent

A   B

The formation of a reentry circuit in WPW syndrome. Current passes down the normal conduction pathways (*A*) and circles back through the bundle of Kent to form a complete reentrant circuit (*B*).

Less commonly, the reentrant mechanism circles the other way, *i.e.*, down the bundle of Kent and back up through the AV node. The result, again, is PSVT, but in this case the QRS complex is wide and bizarre because ventricular depolarization does not occur via the normal bundle branches. This arrhythmia may be indistinguishable from ventricular tachycardia on the EKG.

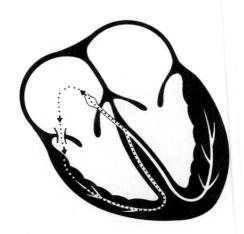

A second type of reentry circuit in WPW syndrome. Current moves antegrade down the bundle of Kent and then retrograde back through the AV node, establishing an independent revolving circuit.

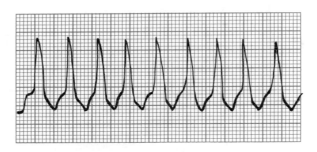

Wide-complex PSVT in WPW syndrome.

In 10% to 15% of patients with WPW, there is more than one accessory pathway, permitting the formation of multiple reentry loops as the current passes up and down through the different Kent bundles and the AV node.

Atrial Fibrillation in WPW

Atrial fibrillation, the other arrhythmia commonly seen in WPW, can be particularly devastating. The bundle of Kent can act as a free conduit for the chaotic atrial activity. Without the AV node to act as a barrier between the atria and ventricles, ventricular rates can rise as high as 300 beats per minute. The precise rate will depend on the refractory period of the bundle of Kent. This rapid atrial fibrillation has been known to induce ventricular fibrillation, a lethal arrhythmia.

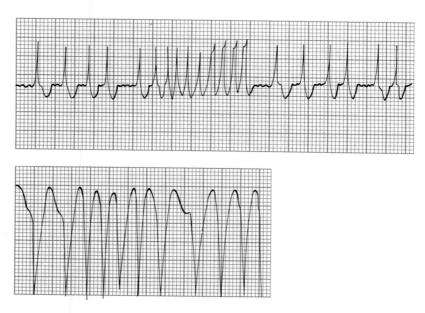

Two examples of atrial fibrillation in WPW syndrome. The ventricular rate is extremely fast.

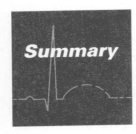

Preexcitation

The diagnosis of preexcitation is made by looking for a short PR interval.

Criteria for WPW Syndrome

1. PR interval less than 0.12 seconds

2. Wide QRS complexes

3. Delta wave seen in some leads.

Criteria for LGL Syndrome

1. PR interval less than 0.12 seconds

2. Normal QRS width

3. No delta wave.

    Arrhythmias commonly seen include the following:

1. Paroxysmal supraventricular tachycardia—narrow QRS complexes are more common than wide ones.

2. Atrial fibrillation—can be very rapid and can lead to ventricular fibrillation.

Note: Because the presence of an accessory pathway in WPW alters the vectors of current flow to at least some degree, you cannot assess axis or amplitude with any precision, and hence any attempt to determine the presence of ventricular hypertrophy or bundle branch block is bound to be unreliable.

Case 6

Winston T., a young investment banker, is brought to the emergency room by his wife when, for no apparent reason at all, he became light-headed and nauseous during dinner. His wife was immediately acquitted when it was learned that Winston was the family chef.

The medical student who is the first to examine him has seen just enough patients to feel overconfident in his diagnostic abilities; tired and overworked, he is ready to send him home with a diagnosis of food poisoning when an astute nurse takes the trouble to put a hand on Winston's pulse and discovers it is extremely rapid. An EKG reveals:

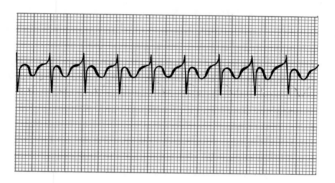

Overcome by his carelessness, the medical student becomes somewhat pallid himself. The emergency room doctor takes over, glances at the rhythm strip and immediately orders a dose of intravenous verapamil. The tachycardia breaks at once and the new rhythm strip looks like this:

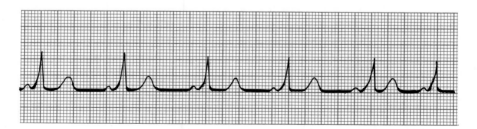

Can you match the emergency room doctor's heady acumen with erudition of your own, and figure out exactly what has happened?

(*continued*)

Winston has Wolff-Parkinson-White syndrome. This is readily apparent from the second EKG, which reveals the characteristic short PR interval, delta wave and prolonged QRS complex. The initial strip shows the typical paroxysmal supraventricular tachycardia that can occur in these individuals. The rapid·tachycardia was responsible for Winston's symptoms, not his admittedly unsavory cooking.

Intravenous verapamil, a calcium channel blocker that can slow electrical conduction through the heart, has proven to be extremely effective at breaking reentrant tachycardias that involve the AV node. This was Winston's first attack, and since most patients with WPW have only infrequent episodes of tachycardia, chronic antiarrhythmic therapy is not indicated at this time.

As for what became of the medical student, he learned from his humiliating experience and went on to become a model of thoroughness and efficiency, eventually graduating at the top of his class. He also has never forgotten the first rule of medicine: **Always take the vital signs.** There is good reason why they are called ''vital.''

The Only EKG Book You'll Ever Need, second edition, by Malcolm S. Thaler.
JB Lippincott Company, Philadelphia © 1995.

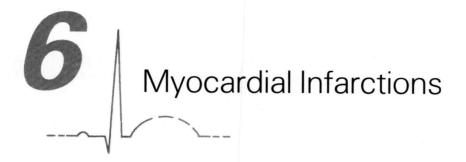

Myocardial Infarctions

In this chapter you will learn:

1 the three things that happen to the EKG during a myocardial infarction (T wave peaking and inversion, ST segment elevation, and the appearance of new Q waves)

2 how to distinguish normal Q waves from the Q waves of infarction

3 how the EKG can localize an infarct to a particular region of the heart

4 the difference between Q wave and non-Q wave infarctions

5 how the EKG changes during an attack of angina (ST segment depression and T wave inversion)

6 how to distinguish typical angina from Prinzmetal's (vasospastic) angina on the EKG

7 the value of stress testing in diagnosing coronary artery disease

8 about the case of Joan L., a woman with an acute infarction and a number of complications requiring your acute attention and incomparable expertise.

⊞ *What Is a Myocardial Infarction?*

A myocardial infarction, or "heart attack," occurs when one of the coronary arteries becomes totally occluded. The region of myocardium supplied by that particular coronary artery loses its blood supply and, deprived of oxygen and other nutrients, dies. The underlying pathogenesis in almost all cases is progressive narrowing of the coronary arteries by atherosclerosis. The sudden, total occlusion that precipitates infarction is usually due to superimposed thrombosis or coronary artery spasm.

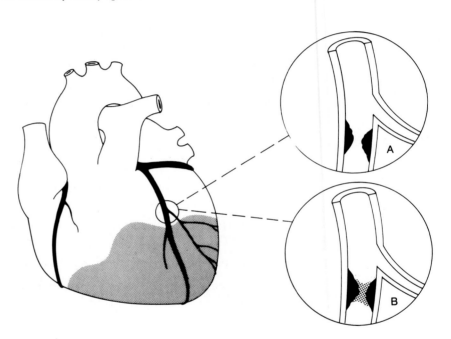

Occlusion of a coronary artery can lead to infarction of the region of myocardium that is dependent on that artery for its blood supply. (*A*) The coronary artery is gradually narrowed by atherosclerotic plaque. (*B*) Infarction can be caused by an acute thrombus superimposed on the underlying plaque.

⊞ *How To Diagnose a Myocardial Infarction*

There are three components to the diagnosis of a myocardial infarction: (1) history and physical examination; (2) cardiac enzyme determinations; and (3) the EKG.

History and Physical Examination. When a patient presents with the typical features of infarction—prolonged, crushing substernal chest pain radiating to the jaw or left arm, associated with nausea, diaphoresis, and shortness of breath—there can be little doubt about the diagnosis. However, many patients, especially those with diabetes mellitus and the elderly, may not manifest all of these symptoms. Some infarctions are even "silent," *i.e.,* they are not associated with any overt clinical manifestations at all.

Cardiac Enzymes. Dying myocardial cells leak their internal contents into the bloodstream. Elevated blood levels of creatine kinase (CK), lactic dehydrogenase (LDH), and aspartate aminotransferase (or serum glutamic-oxaloacetic transaminase [SGOT]) are strongly indicative of an infarction. However, these enzymes require several hours to achieve diagnostic blood levels, and it is important to diagnose a myocardial infarction as quickly as possible.

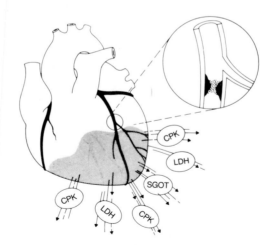

Intracellular enzymes are released by the dying myocardial cells after complete coronary occlusion results in acute infarction.

The EKG. In the vast majority of infarctions, the EKG will reveal the correct diagnosis. Characteristic electrocardiographic changes accompany myocardial infarction, and the earliest changes occur almost at once with the onset of myocardial compromise. An EKG should be performed immediately in any person in whom an infarction is even remotely suspected. However, the initial EKG may not always be diagnostic, and the evolution of electrocardiographic changes varies from person to person, so it is necessary to obtain serial cardiograms once the patient is admitted to the hospital.

Rarely, all three of these components fail to establish the diagnosis with certainty. Special studies can then be performed in an attempt to firm up or rule out the diagnosis of infarction. The most widely used of these is radioactive technetium labeling. Technetium binds to regions of damaged myocardium, which will then light up on scanning. Newer and possibly more sensitive tests, such as labeled antibodies that bind to various components of cardiac muscle, are under study.

During an acute myocardial infarction, the EKG evolves through three stages:

1. T wave peaking followed by T wave inversion (**A** and **B**, below)

2. ST segment elevation (**C**)

3. Appearance of new Q waves (**D**).

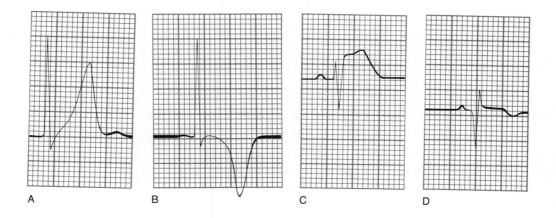

A   B   C   D

> Although the EKG does typically evolve through these three stages during an acute infarction, any one of these changes may be present without any of the others. Thus, for example, it is not at all unusual to see ST segment elevation without T wave inversion, as in figure **C** above. Learn to recognize each of these three changes, keep your suspicion of myocardial infarction high, and you will never go wrong.

The T Wave

With the onset of infarction the T waves become tall and narrow, a phenomenon called *peaking*. These peaked T waves are often referred to as *hyperacute T waves*. Shortly afterward, usually a few hours later, the T waves invert.

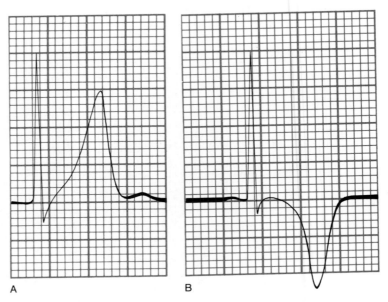

(*A*) T wave peaking in a patient undergoing acute infarction. (*B*) The same lead in a patient 2 hours later shows T wave inversion.

These T wave changes reflect myocardial *ischemia*, the lack of adequate blood flow to the myocardium.

Ischemia is potentially reversible: if blood flow is restored or the oxygen demands of the heart are eased, the T waves will revert to normal. On the other hand, if actual myocardial cell death (true infarction) has occurred, T wave inversion will persist for months to years.

T wave inversion by itself is indicative only of ischemia and is not diagnostic of myocardial infarction.

T wave inversion is a very nonspecific finding. Many things can cause a T wave to flip; for example, we have already seen that both bundle branch block and ventricular hypertrophy with strain are associated with T wave inversion.

One helpful diagnostic feature is that the T waves of myocardial ischemia are inverted *symmetrically,* whereas in most other circumstances they are asymmetric, with a gentle downslope and rapid upslope.

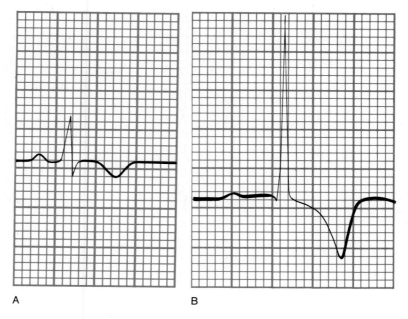

A   B

(*A*) The symmetric T wave inversion in a patient with ischemia. (*B*) An example of asymmetric T wave inversion in a patient with left ventricular hypertrophy and strain.

In patients whose T waves are already inverted, ischemia may cause them to revert to normal, a phenomenon called *pseudonormalization.* Recognition of pseudonormalization requires comparing the current EKG with a previous tracing.

The ST Segment

ST segment elevation is the second change that occurs acutely in the evolution of an infarction.

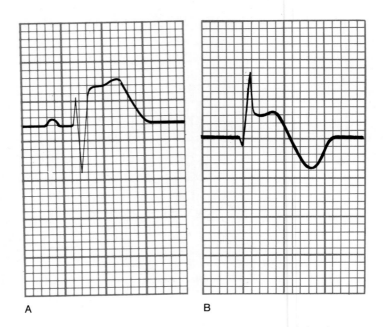

Two examples of ST segment elevation during an acute infarction:
(*A*) Without T wave inversion and (*B*) with T wave inversion.

ST segment elevation signifies myocardial *injury*. Injury probably reflects a degree of cellular damage beyond that of mere ischemia, but it, too, is potentially reversible, and in some cases the ST segments may rapidly return to normal. In most instances, however, ST segment elevation is a reliable sign that true infarction has occurred and that the complete electrocardiographic picture of infarction will evolve.

Even in the setting of a true infarction, the ST segments usually return to baseline within a few hours. Persistent ST segment elevation often indicates the formation of a *ventricular aneurysm*, a weakening and bulging of the ventricular wall.

Like T wave inversion, ST segment elevation can be seen in a number of other conditions in addition to myocardial injury. There is even a type of ST segment elevation that can be seen in normal hearts. This phenomenon has been referred to as *early repolarization* (actually a physiologic misnomer) or *J point elevation* (a much better term). The *J point*, or *junction point*, is the place where the ST segment takes off from the QRS complex.

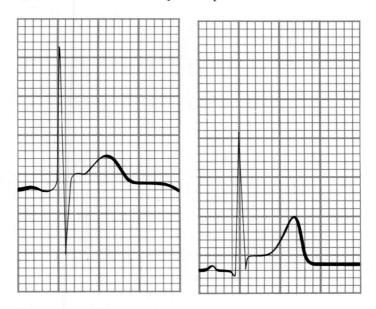

Two examples of J point elevation.

J point elevation is very common in young, healthy individuals. The ST segment usually returns to baseline with exercise. J point elevation has no pathologic implications whatsoever.

How can the ST segment elevation of myocardial injury be distinguished from that of J point elevation? With myocardial disease, the elevated ST segment has a distinctive configuration. It is bowed upward and tends to merge imperceptibly with the T wave. In J point elevation, the T wave maintains its independent waveform.

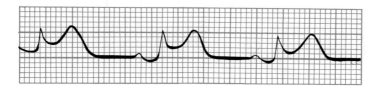

ST segment elevation during an infarction. Note how the ST segment and T wave merge into each other without a clear demarcation between them.

Q Waves

The appearance of new Q waves indicates that irreversible myocardial cell death has occurred. The presence of Q waves is diagnostic of myocardial infarction.

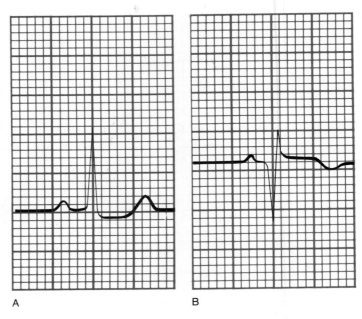

A   B

(*A*) Lead III in a healthy patient. (*B*) The same lead in the same patient 2 weeks after undergoing an inferior myocardial infarction. Note the deep Q wave.

Q waves usually appear within several hours of the onset of infarction, but in some patients they may take several days to evolve. The ST segment usually has returned to baseline by the time Q waves have appeared. Q waves tend to persist for the lifetime of the patient.

Why Q Waves Form

The genesis of Q waves as a sign of infarction is easy to understand. When a region of myocardium dies, it becomes electrically silent—it is no longer able to conduct an electrical current. As a result, all of the electrical forces of the heart will be directed *away* from the area of infarction. An electrode overlying the infarct will therefore record a deep negative deflection, a Q wave.

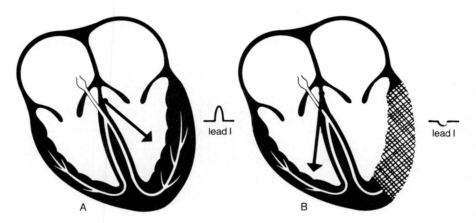

(*A*) Normal left ventricular depolarization with the arrow showing the electrical axis. Note the tall R wave in lead I. (*B*) The lateral wall of the left ventricle has infarcted, and, as a result, is now electrically silent. The electrical axis therefore shifts rightward, away from lead I, which now shows a negative deflection (Q wave).

Reciprocal Changes

Other leads, located some distance from the site of infarction, will see an apparent increase in the electrical forces moving toward them. They will record tall positive R waves.

These opposing changes seen by distant leads are called *reciprocal changes*. The concept of reciprocity applies not only to Q waves but also to ST segment and T wave changes. Thus, a lead distant from an infarct may record ST segment *depression*.

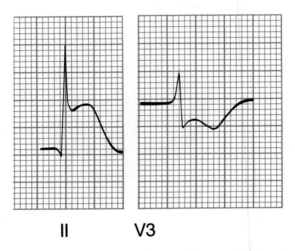

II   V3

Reciprocal changes in an inferior infarction. The acute ST elevation and T wave peaking in lead II is echoed by the ST depression and T wave inversion in lead V_3.

Normal Versus Pathologic Q Waves

Small Q waves can be seen in the left lateral leads (I, AVL, V₅, and V₆) and occasionally in the inferior leads (especially II and III) of perfectly normal hearts. These Q waves are caused by the early left-to-right depolarization of the interventricular septum.

Pathologic Q waves signifying infarction tend to be *wider* and *deeper*. They are often referred to as *significant Q waves*. The criteria for significance are

1. The Q wave must be greater than 0.04 seconds in duration.

2. The depth of the Q wave must be at least one-third the height of the R wave in the same QRS complex.

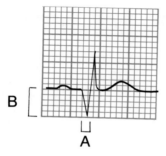

An example of a significant Q wave. Its width (*A*) exceeds 0.04 seconds and its depth (*B*) exceeds one-third that of the R wave.

Note: Because lead AVR occupies a unique position on the frontal plane, it normally has a very deep Q wave. Lead AVR should *not* be considered when assessing possible infarction.

Are the following Q waves significant?

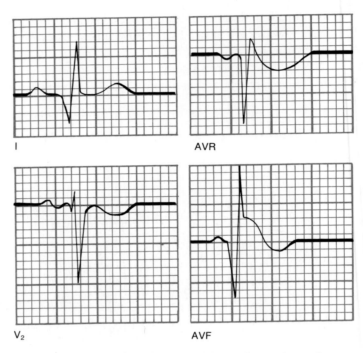

Answers: The Q waves in leads I and AVF are significant. The Q wave
in lead V₂ is too shallow and narrow to qualify. The Q wave in lead AVR
is immense, but Q waves in AVR are never significant!

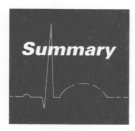

Summary

The EKG Changes of an Evolving Myocardial Infarction

1. Acutely, the T wave peaks and then inverts. T wave changes reflect myocardial ischemia. If true infarction occurs, the T wave remains inverted for months to years.

2. Acutely, the ST segment elevates and merges with the T wave. ST segment elevation reflects myocardial injury. If infarction occurs, the ST segment usually returns to baseline within a few hours.

3. New Q waves appear within hours to days. They signify myocardial infarction. In most cases, they persist for the lifetime of the patient.

Today, it is critical to recognize a myocardial infarction as early as possible. Medications can be given intravenously in the emergency room to actually *prevent* the completion of the infarction if they are given within the first few hours of the onset of the attack. By the time Q waves have formed, it may be too late to intervene.

These medications are thrombolytic agents, capable of lysing a clot within the coronary arteries and thereby reestablishing blood flow before myocardial death has occurred. The three most common agents in use are streptokinase, anisoylated plasminogen activator complex, and tissue plasminogen activator. Which one is the best? Studies show that they are essentially equivalent, and that each conveys a substantial survival benefit as long as it is given within 12 hours of the onset of symptoms. Therefore, your ability to recognize promptly the early T wave and ST segment changes on the EKG could save a life.

⊞ *Localizing the Infarct*

The region of myocardium that undergoes infarction depends on which coronary artery becomes occluded and the extent of collateral blood flow. There are two major systems of blood supply to the myocardium, one supplying the right side of the heart and one supplying the left side.

The *right coronary artery* runs between the right atrium and right ventricle and then swings around to the posterior surface of the heart. In most individuals, it gives off a descending branch that supplies the AV node.

The *left main artery* divides into a *left anterior descending artery (LAD)* and a *left circumflex artery*. The LAD supplies the anterior wall of the heart and most of the interventricular septum. The circumflex artery runs between the left atrium and left ventricle and supplies the lateral wall of the left ventricle. In about 10% of the population it gives off the branch that supplies the AV node.

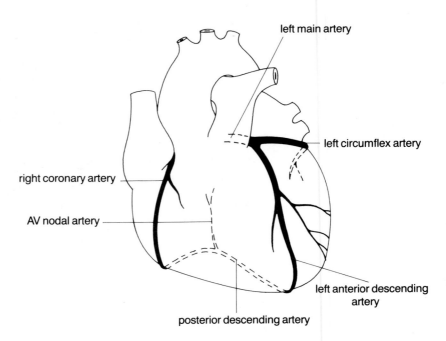

The main coronary arteries.

Localization of an infarct is important, because the prognostic and therapeutic implications are largely determined by which area of the heart has died.

Infarctions can be grouped into several general anatomic categories. These are inferior infarctions, lateral wall infarctions, anterior infarctions, and posterior infarctions. Combinations can also be seen, *e.g.* anterolateral infarctions, which are most common.

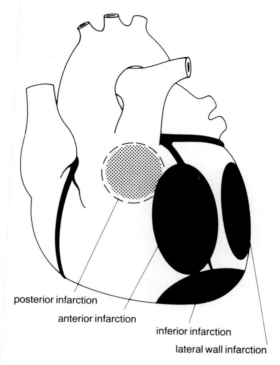

posterior infarction

anterior infarction

inferior infarction

lateral wall infarction

The four basic anatomical sites of myocardial infarction.

Almost all myocardial infarctions involve the left ventricle. This should not be surprising, because the left ventricle is the most muscular chamber and is called on to do the most work. It is therefore most vulnerable to a compromised blood supply. Some inferior infarctions also involve a portion of the right ventricle.

The characteristic electrocardiographic changes of infarction occur only in those leads overlying or near the site of infarction.

1. *Inferior infarction* involves the diaphragmatic surface of the heart. It is often caused by occlusion of the right coronary artery or its descending branch. The characteristic electrocardiographic changes of infarction can be seen in the inferior leads II, III, and AVF.

2. *Lateral wall infarction* involves the left lateral wall of the heart. It is often due to occlusion of the left circumflex artery. Changes will occur in the left lateral leads I, AVL, V_5, and V_6.

3. *Anterior infarction* involves the anterior surface of the left ventricle and is usually caused by occlusion of the left anterior descending artery. Any of the precordial leads (V_1 through V_6) may show changes.

4. *Posterior infarction* involves the posterior surface of the heart and is usually caused by occlusion of the right coronary artery. There are no leads overlying the posterior wall. The diagnosis must therefore be made by looking for reciprocal changes in the anterior leads, especially V_1. This will be discussed later.

Actually, it is a very simple matter to put electrodes on a patient's back to get a good look at the posterior electrical forces. When this is done (and, unfortunately, it is done only rarely), the ability of the EKG to diagnose a myocardial infarction is greatly enhanced. These so-called 15-lead EKGs, which include two V leads placed on the back (V_8 and V_9) and one on the right anterior chest wall (V_{4R}) have been found to detect ST segment elevation in many patients with suspected infarction in whom the 12-lead EKG is normal.

Note: Coronary anatomy can vary markedly among individuals, and the precise vessel involved may not always be what one would predict from the EKG.

Inferior Infarcts

Inferior infarction typically results from occlusion of the right coronary artery or its descending branch. Changes occur in leads II, III, and AVF. Reciprocal changes may be seen in the anterior and left lateral leads.

Although in most infarctions significant Q waves persist for the lifetime of the patient, this is not necessarily true with inferior infarcts. Within half a year as many as 50% of these patients will lose their criteria for significant Q waves. The presence of small Q waves inferiorly may therefore suggest an old inferior infarction. Remember, however, that small inferior Q waves also may be seen in normal hearts. The clinical history of the patient must be your guide.

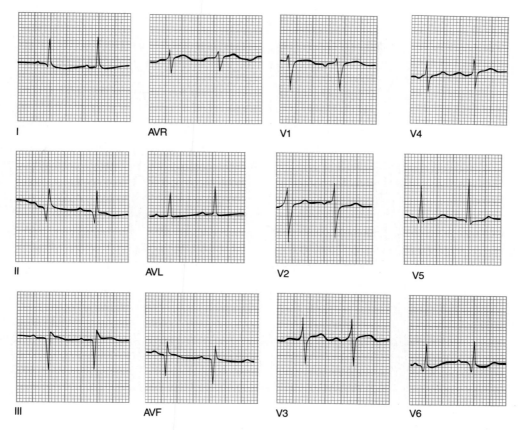

A fully evolved inferior infarction. Deep Q waves can be seen in leads II, III, and AVF.

Lateral Wall Infarction

Lateral wall infarction may result from occlusion of the left circumflex artery. Changes may be seen in leads I, AVL, V_5, and V_6. Reciprocal changes may be seen in the inferior leads.

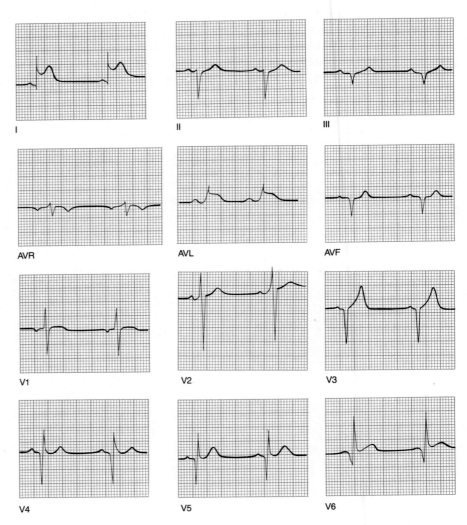

An acute lateral wall infarction. ST elevation can be seen in leads I, AVL, V_5, and V_6. Note also the deep Q waves in leads II, III, and AVF, signifying a previous inferior infarction.

Anterior Infarcts

Anterior infarction may result from occlusion of the LAD. Changes are seen in the precordial leads (V_1 through V_6). If the left main artery is occluded, an anterolateral infarction may result, with changes in the precordial leads and in leads I and AVL. Reciprocal changes are seen inferiorly.

The loss of anterior electrical forces in anterior infarction is not always associated with Q wave formation. In some patients, there may be only a loss or diminishment of the normal pattern of precordial R wave progression. As you already know, under normal circumstances the precordial leads show a progressive increase in the height of each successive R wave as one moves from V_1 to V_5. This pattern may vanish with anterior infarction, and the result is called *poor R wave progression.* Even in the absence of significant Q waves, poor R wave progression may signify an anterior infarction.

Poor R wave progression is not specific for the diagnosis of anterior infarction. It also can be seen with right ventricular hypertrophy, in patients with chronic lung disease, and—perhaps most often—with improper lead placement.

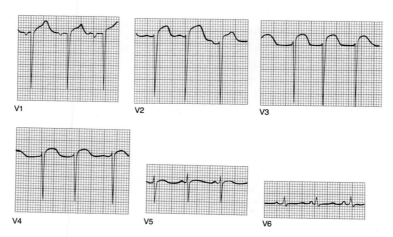

An anterior infarction with poor R wave progression across the precordium.

Posterior Infarction

Posterior infarction typically results from an occlusion of the right coronary artery. Since no leads overlie the posterior wall, the diagnosis requires finding reciprocal changes in the anterior leads. In other words, since we can't look for ST segment elevation and Q waves in nonexistent posterior leads, we have to look for *ST segment depression* and *tall R waves* in the anterior leads, notably lead V_1. Posterior infarctions are the mirror images of anterior infarctions on the EKG.

The normal QRS complex in lead V_1 consists of a small R wave and a deep S wave, so the presence of a tall R wave, particularly with accompanying ST segment depression, should be easy to spot. In the appropriate clinical setting, the presence of an R wave of greater amplitude than the corresponding S wave is highly suggestive of a posterior infarction.

Another helpful clue comes from the blood supply of the heart. Because the inferior wall usually has the same blood supply as the posterior wall, there will often be evidence of accompanying infarction of the inferior wall.

One caveat: You will recall (no doubt) that the presence of a large R wave exceeding the amplitude of the accompanying S wave in lead V_1 is also one criterion for the diagnosis of right ventricular hypertrophy. The diagnosis of right ventricular hypertrophy, however, also requires the presence of right axis deviation, which is not present in posterior infarction.

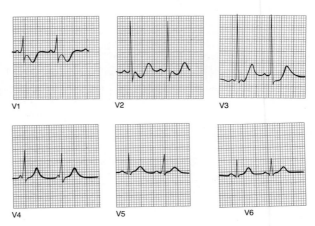

A posterior infarction. In lead V_1, the R wave is larger than the S wave. There is also ST depression and T wave inversion in leads V_1 and V_2.

Where is the infarct? Is it acute?

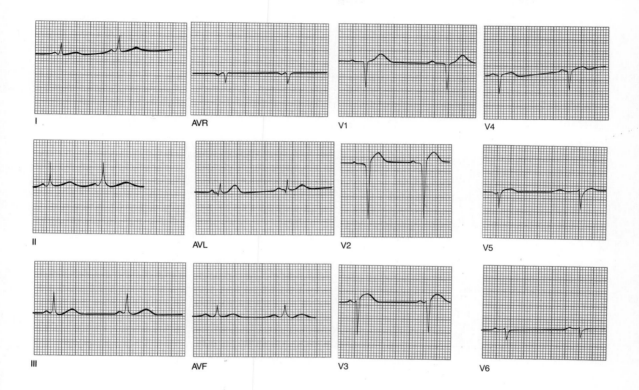

I   AVR   V1   V4

II   AVL   V2   V5

III   AVF   V3   V6

This is an example of an evolving anterior infarction. There is ST segment elevation in leads V_2 and V_3, as well as poor R wave progression.

Where is the infarct? Is it acute?

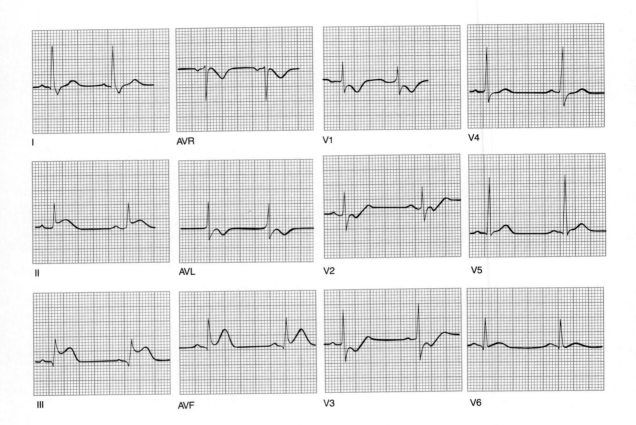

This tracing shows an acute posterior and inferior infarction (remember now we said that most posterior infarctions are accompanied by evidence of inferior infarction?). ST segment elevation with peaked T waves can be seen in leads II, III, and AVF, indicating an acute inferior infarction. There is also evidence of posterior wall involvement, with a tall R wave, ST segment depression and T wave inversion in lead V_1.

⊞ Non–Q Wave Myocardial Infarctions

Not all myocardial infarctions produce Q waves. It was previously thought that the production of Q waves required infarction of the entire thickness of the myocardial wall, whereas an absence of Q waves indicated infarction of only a portion of the inner layer of the myocardial wall called the subendocardium. People therefore spoke of infarctions as being transmural or subendocardial.

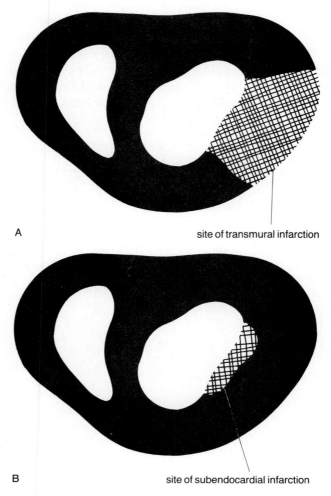

A

site of transmural infarction

B

site of subendocardial infarction

(A) Depiction of a transmural infarction and (B) a subendocardial infarction.

However, pathologic studies have found little consistent correlation between the evolution of Q waves and whether an infarction is transmural or subendocardial. Some transmural infarctions fail to produce Q waves, and some subendocardial infarctions do produce Q waves. For this reason, the old terminology, however descriptive, has been dropped and replaced by the far less picturesque terms "Q wave infarctions" and "non–Q wave infarctions."

The only EKG changes seen with non–Q wave infarctions are T wave inversion and ST segment depression.

We do know that non–Q wave infarctions do have a lower initial mortality rate and a higher risk of later infarction and mortality than do Q wave infarctions. Non-Q wave infarctions seem to behave like small, incomplete infarctions, and cardiologists take a very aggressive stance with these patients, evaluating them thoroughly and intervening therapeutically (with either traditional coronary bypass grafting or any of the various angioplasty procedures now in vogue) in an effort to prevent further infarction and death.

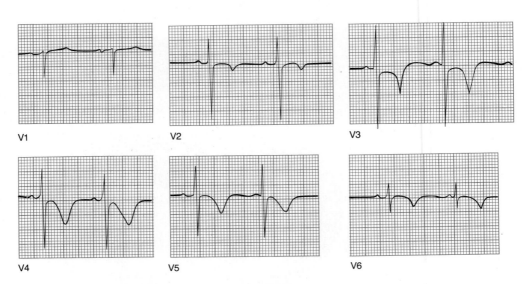

A non-Q wave infarction. ST segment depression is most prominent in leads V_2 and V_3, and T wave inversion can be seen in leads V_2 through V_6. This patient never evolved Q waves, but his cardiac enzymes soared, confirming occurrence of a true infarction.

⊞ *Angina*

Angina is the typical chest pain associated with coronary artery disease. A patient with angina may ultimately go on to experience an infarction or may remain stable for many years. An EKG taken during an anginal attack will show *ST segment depression* or *T wave inversion*.

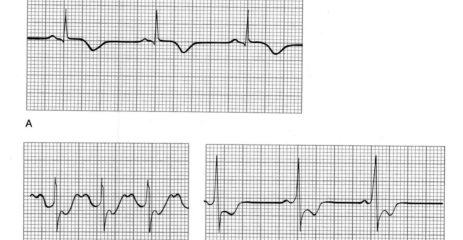

A

B   C

Three examples of the EKG changes that can accompany angina: (*A*) T wave inversion; (*B*) ST segment depression; and (*C*) ST segment depression with T wave inversion.

The two ways to distinguish the ST segment depression of angina from that of non–Q wave infarctions are the clinical picture and the time course. With angina, the ST segments usually return to baseline shortly after the attack has subsided. With a non–Q wave infarction, the ST segments remain down for at least 48 hours. Cardiac enzyme determinations can be helpful because they will be elevated with infarction but not with uncomplicated angina.

Prinzmetal's Angina

There is one type of angina that is associated with ST segment *elevation*. Whereas typical angina is usually brought on by exertion and is the result of progressive atherosclerotic cardiovascular disease, Prinzmetal's angina can occur at any time and in many patients is due to coronary artery spasm. Presumably, the ST segment elevation reflects reversible transmural injury. The contours of the ST segments often will not have the rounded, domed appearance of true infarction, and the ST segments will return quickly to baseline when the patient is given antianginal medication (e.g. nitroglycerin).

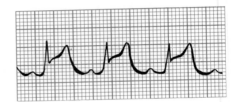

Prinzmetal's angina, with ST segment elevation.

Patients with Prinzmetal's angina actually fall into two groups: those with no atherosclerotic disease whose pain is due solely to coronary artery spasm, and those with some underlying atherosclerotic disease who may or may not have superimposed spasm. The EKG does not help to distinguish between these two groups.

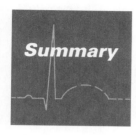

The ST Segment in Cardiac Disease

ST Segment Elevation

May be seen with an evolving transmural infarction or with Prinzmetal's angina

ST Segment Depression

May be seen with typical angina or with a non–Q wave infarction

⊞ *Limitations of the EKG in Diagnosing an Infarction*

The electrocardiographic picture of an evolving transmural myocardial infarction includes ST segment changes and the appearance of new Q waves. Any underlying cardiac condition that masks these effects by distorting the ST segment and QRS complex will render electrocardiographic diagnosis of an infarction impossible. Two such conditions are Wolff-Parkinson-White syndrome and left bundle branch block. Right bundle branch block is of less concern because almost all infarctions involve the left ventricle.

Rule: In the presence of left bundle branch block or Wolff-Parkinson-White syndrome, the diagnosis of a myocardial infarction cannot be reliably made by EKG.

⊞ *Stress Testing*

Stress testing, also called exercise tolerance testing, is a noninvasive method of assessing the presence and severity of coronary artery disease. It is by no means flawless (false-positives and false-negatives abound), but it is the best screening procedure available. The alternative—taking all candidates directly to cardiac catheterization—is neither feasible nor desirable.

Stress testing is usually done by having the patient ambulate on a treadmill, although stationary bicycles have been used just as effectively. The patient is hooked up to an EKG monitor and a rhythm strip is run continuously through-out the test. A complete 12-lead EKG is taken at frequent intervals. Every few minutes the speed and angle of incline of the treadmill are increased until (1) the patient cannot continue for whatever reason; (2) the patient's maximal heart rate is achieved; (3) symptoms supervene; or (4) significant changes are seen on the EKG.

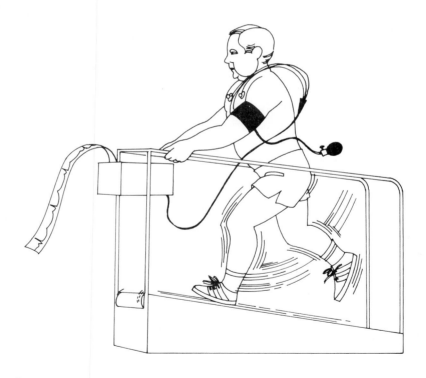

The physiology behind stress testing is simple. The graded exercise protocol causes a safe and gradual increase in the patient's heart rate and systolic blood pressure. The product of the patient's blood pressure multiplied by his heart rate, called the *double product,* is a good measure of myocardial oxygen consumption. If cardiac oxygen demands exceed consumption, electrocardiographic changes (and sometimes symptoms) of myocardial ischemia may occur.

Significant coronary artery disease of one or several coronary arteries limits blood flow to the myocardium and hence limits oxygen consumption. Although the resting EKG may be normal, the increased demands of exercise may bring out evidence of subclinical coronary artery disease.

With a positive test for coronary artery disease, the EKG will reveal *ST segment depression.* T wave changes are too nonspecific to have any meaning in this setting.

There is a wealth of literature questioning precisely what constitutes significant ST segment depression during an exercise test. It is generally acknowledged that ST segment depression of greater than 1 mm that is horizontal or downsloping and persists for more than 0.08 seconds is suggestive of coronary artery disease. If a depression of 2 mm is used as the criterion, the number of false-positives is greatly reduced but the number of false-negatives increases. Occasionally, upsloping ST segments may signify coronary artery disease, but the number of false-positives is very high.

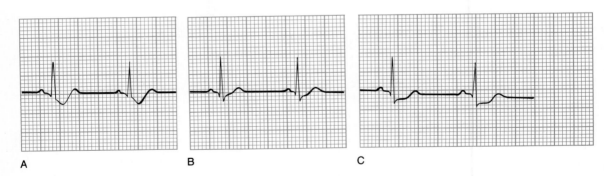

A   B   C

(A) Downsloping ST depression. (B) Upsloping ST depression. (C) Horizontal ST depression. Only A and C are highly suggestive of coronary artery disease.

The earlier in the test that ST segment depression occurs, particularly if the changes persist several minutes into the recovery period, the greater the likelihood that coronary artery disease is present, and the greater the possibility that the left main coronary artery or several coronary arteries are involved. The onset of symptoms or a falling blood pressure are particularly important signs, and the test must be stopped immediately.

The incidence of false-positives and false-negatives is dependent on the patient population that is being tested. A positive test in a young healthy individual with no symptoms and no risk factors for coronary artery disease is likely to be a false test. On the other hand, a positive test in an elderly man with chest pain, a prior infarction, and hypertension is much more likely to be a true-positive. In no one does a negative test absolutely exclude the possibility of coronary artery disease.

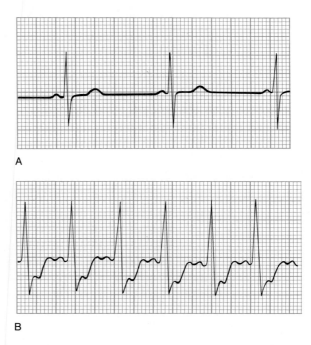

(*A*) A patient's resting EKG. (*B*) The same lead in the same patient 12 minutes into an exercise test. Note the prominent ST segment depression associated with the increased heart rate.

Indications for stress testing include the following:

1. The differential diagnosis of chest pain in someone whose baseline EKG is normal

2. The evaluation of a patient who has recently had an infarction, in order to assess his prognosis and need for further invasive testing, such as cardiac catheterization

3. The general evaluation of individuals over 40 years of age who have risk factors for coronary artery disease. The indications for stress testing in this population are less clear-cut. Stress testing is also frequently done in patients over 40 years of age who want to start an exercise program.

Contraindications include any acute systemic illness, severe aortic stenosis, uncontrolled congestive heart failure, severe hypertension, angina at rest, and the presence of a significant arrhythmia.

Mortality from the procedure is very low, but resuscitation equipment should always be available.

Both the sensitivity and specificity of the exercise stress test can be increased by approximately 15% by injecting the patient with radioactive thallium-201 during the test and then imaging the heart several minutes later. The myocardium extracts the radiotracer from the coronary circulation, but regions of compromised blood flow will be unable to extract the radiotracer. Therefore, in a normal test, myocardial scintigraphy will reveal uniform uptake of the thallium-201 by the left ventricle, but in a patient with coronary stenosis a large perfusion defect may be seen. Some time later, a second film is taken, at which point the heart is no longer under stress. The perfusion defect may now disappear, indicating that the stenosed coronary artery is supplying blood to viable myocardium; medical or surgical intervention to treat the stenosis may therefore preserve the affected region of the left ventricle. On the other hand, if the perfusion defect does not disappear on the second film, one can conclude that the region in question is no longer metabolically capable of taking up the tracer, and is therefore most likely infarcted; restoring blood flow to that region of the heart is unlikely to be of any benefit.

Case 7

Joan L. is a 62-year-old business executive. She is on an important business trip and spends the night at a hotel downtown. Early the next morning she is awakened with shortness of breath and severe chest pressure that radiates into her jaw and left arm. She gets out of bed and takes Pepto-Bismol, but the pain does not go away. Feeling somewhat dizzy and nauseous, she sits down and phones the front desk. Her symptoms are relayed by phone to the doctor covering the hotel, who immediately orders an ambulance to take her to the local emergency room. She arrives there only 2 hours after the onset of her symptoms, which have continued unabated despite three sublingual nitroglycerin given to her during the ambulance ride.

In the emergency room, a 12-lead EKG reveals the following. Is she having an infarction? If so, can you tell if it is acute and what region of the heart is affected?

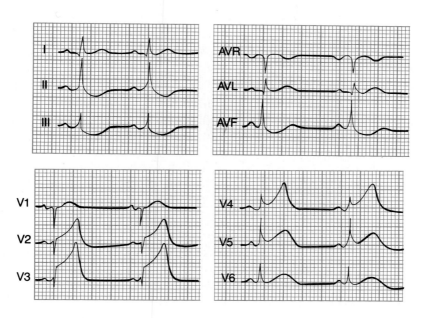

(continued)

The EKG shows ST segment elevation in leads V_2 through V_5. There are no Q waves. Joan is in the throes of an acute anterior myocardial infarction.

Joan's prompt arrival in the emergency room and absence of Q waves on the EKG mean that she is an excellent candidate for thrombolytic therapy. Unfortunately, she relates that only one month ago she suffered a mild stroke, leaving her with some weakness in her left arm and leg. After much fevered discussion, it is decided that the risk of thrombolytic therapy causing an intracerebral bleed outweighs the potential benefits. Thrombolytic therapy is withheld, and Joan is taken to the cardiac care unit (CCU) to be monitored.

Late on the first night of her hospital stay, one of the nurses notices peculiar beats on her EKG. What are they?

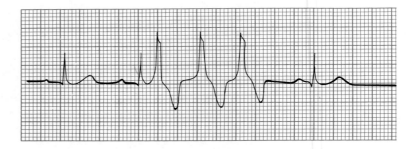

The patient's normal sinus rhythm is being interrupted by frequent PVCs, including one run of three consecutive PVCs. In the setting of an acute infarction, lidocaine must be given immediately because these PVCs can trigger ventricular tachycardia and fibrillation.

The next morning, Joan's EKG looks like this. What has changed?

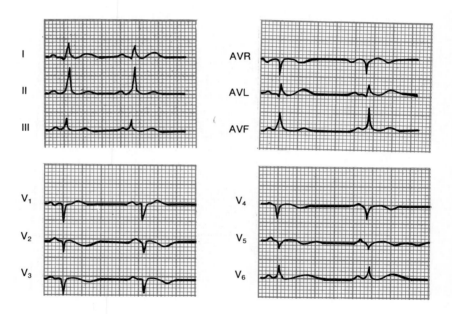

(continued)

Joan's EKG shows that all ventricular ectopy has been suppressed. It also shows new Q waves in the anterior leads, consistent with full evolution of an anterior infarct. Cardiac enzyme determinations would probably be very high.

Later in the afternoon, Joan begins to experience chest pain. A repeat EKG is taken. What has changed?

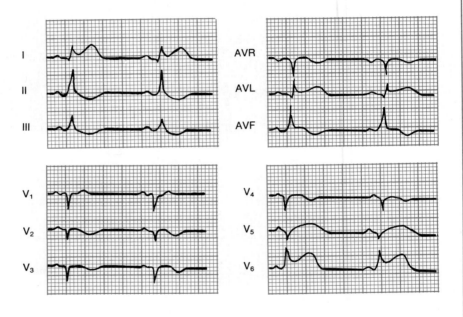

Joan is extending her infarct. New ST elevations can be seen in the left lateral leads.

A few hours later she complains of light-headedness, and another EKG is performed. Now what do you see?

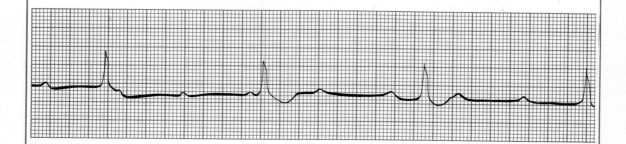

(continued)

Joan has gone into third-degree AV block. Serious conduction blocks are commonly seen in anterior infarctions. Her light-headedness is due to inadequate cardiac output in the face of a ventricular escape rhythm of approximately 35 beats per minute. Pacemaker insertion is mandatory.

A pacemaker is placed without difficulty and Joan suffers no further complications during her hospital stay. One week later, ambulatory and pain-free, she is discharged. The morning after returning home, she again awakens short of breath, and is taken to the emergency room. There she is found to be in congestive heart failure. A cardiac echogram reveals markedly diminished left ventricular function as a result of her large myocardial infarction. She is treated in the hospital and is discharged three days later on a diuretic and vasodilator. No further problems develop, and she is able to return to her normal life at home and at work.

This case is very typical of the sort of thing you see over and over again in hospitals across the country. It emphasizes how critical the EKG still is in diagnosing and managing patients with acute myocardial infarctions. With Joan, an EKG confirmed the initial suspicion that she was having an infarct. In the CCU, electrocardiographic surveillance permitted the diagnosis of further infarction and accompanying rhythm and conduction disturbances, and guided major therapeutic decisions.

The Only EKG Book You'll Ever Need, second edition, by Malcolm S. Thaler. JB Lippincott Company, Philadelphia © 1995.

Finishing Touches

In this chapter you will learn:

1 that the EKG can be changed by a whole variety of other cardiac and noncardiac disorders, most particularly:

    a electrolyte disturbances

    b hypothermia

    c drugs

    d other cardiac disorders (*e.g.,* pericarditis, cardiomyopathy, and myocarditis)

    e pulmonary disorders

    f central nervous system disease

    g athletic activity

2 about the case of Amos T., whose EKG proves to be the key to unravelling an emergent, life-threatening noncardiac condition.

There are a number of medications, electrolyte disturbances, and other disorders that can substantially alter the normal pattern of the EKG. It is not always clear *why* the EKG is so sensitive to such a seemingly diffuse array of conditions, but it is, and you've got to know about them.

In some of these instances, the EKG may actually be the most sensitive indicator of impending catastrophe. In others, subtle electrocardiographic changes may be an early clue to a previously unsuspected problem. In still others, the electrocardiographic alteration may be incidental, vaguely interesting, and hardly illuminating.

We will not dwell on mechanisms in this chapter. In many cases the reasons behind the changes in the EKG simply are not known. The topics we shall cover include the following:

- Electrolyte disturbances
- Hypothermia
- Drugs
- Other cardiac disorders
- Pulmonary disorders
- Central nervous system disease
- The athlete's heart.

⊞ *Electrolyte Disturbances*

Alterations in the serum levels of potassium and calcium can profoundly alter the EKG.

Hyperkalemia

Hyperkalemia produces a progressive evolution of changes in the EKG that can culminate in ventricular fibrillation and death. The presence of electrocardiographic changes is probably a better measure of clinically significant potassium toxicity than the serum potassium level.

1. As the potassium begins to rise, the T waves across the entire 12-lead EKG begin to peak. This effect can easily be confused with the peaked T waves of an acute myocardial infarction. One difference is that the changes in an infarction are confined to those leads overlying the area of the infarct, whereas in hyperkalemia the changes are diffuse.

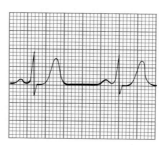

The peaked T waves of hyperkalemia.

2. With a further increase in the serum potassium, the PR interval becomes prolonged and the P wave gradually flattens and then disappears.

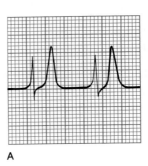

A

(A) As the potassium level rises, P waves are no longer visible. The T waves are even more peaked.

3. Ultimately, the QRS complex widens until it merges with the T wave, forming a *sine wave* pattern. Ventricular fibrillation may eventually develop.

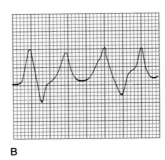

B

(B) Progressive hyperkalemia leads to the classic sine wave pattern. The widened QRS complexes and peaked T waves are almost indistinguishable.

It is important to note that, whereas these changes frequently do occur in the order described as the serum potassium rises, they do not *always* do so. Progression to ventricular fibrillation can occur with devastating suddenness. **Any change in the EKG due to hyperkalemia mandates immediate clinical attention!**

Hypokalemia

With hypokalemia, the EKG may again be a better measure of serious toxicity than the serum potassium level. Three changes can be seen, occurring in no particular order:

- ST segment depression

- Flattening of the T wave

- Appearance of a U wave.

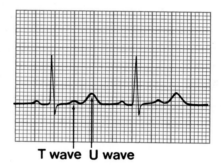

T wave U wave

Hypokalemia. The U waves are even more prominent than the T waves.

The term *U wave* is given to a wave appearing after the T wave in the cardiac cycle. Its precise physiologic meaning is not fully understood. Although U waves are the most characteristic feature of hypokalemia, they are not in and of themselves diagnostic. Other conditions can produce prominent U waves, and U waves can sometimes be seen in patients with normal hearts and normal serum potassium levels.

Calcium Disorders

Alterations in the serum calcium primarily affect the QT interval. Hypocalcemia prolongs it; hypercalcemia shortens it. Do you remember a potentially lethal arrhythmia associated with a prolonged QT interval?

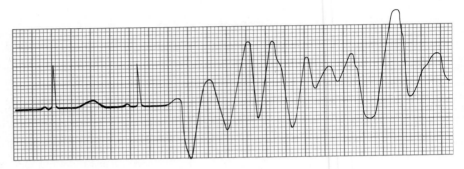

Hypocalcemia. The QT interval is slightly prolonged. A PVC falls on the prolonged T wave and sets off a run of torsades de pointes.

Torsades de pointes, a variant of ventricular tachycardia, is seen in patients with prolonged QT intervals.

⊞ *Hypothermia*

As the body temperature dips below 30°C, several changes occur on the EKG:

1. Everything slows down. Sinus bradycardia is common, and all the intervals—PR, QRS, QT—may become prolonged.

2. A distinctive and virtually diagnostic type of ST segment elevation may be seen. It consists of an abrupt ascent right at the J point and then an equally sudden plunge back to baseline. The resultant configuration is called a *J wave* or *Osborne wave.*

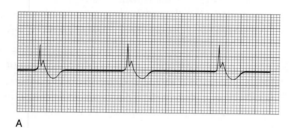

A

(*A*) Hypothermia. The Osborne waves are very prominent.

3. Various arrhythmias may ultimately supervene. Slow atrial fibrillation is most common, although almost any rhythm disturbance can occur.

4. A muscle tremor artifact due to shivering may complicate the tracing. A similar artifact may be seen in patients with Parkinson's disease. Do not confuse this with atrial flutter.

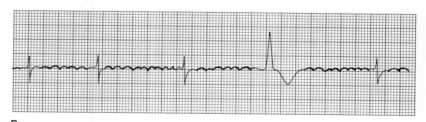

B

(*B*) A muscle tremor artifact resembles atrial flutter.

⊞ *Drugs*

Digitalis

There are two distinct categories of electrocardiographic alterations caused by digitalis: those associated with *therapeutic* blood levels of the drug, and those seen with *toxic* blood levels.

EKG Changes Associated With Therapeutic Blood Levels

Therapeutic levels of digitalis produce characteristic ST segment and T wave changes in most individuals taking the drug. These changes are known as the *digitalis effect* and consist of ST segment depression with flattening or inversion of the T wave. The depressed ST segments have a very gradual downslope, emerging almost imperceptibly from the preceding R wave. This distinctive appearance usually permits differentiation of the digitalis effect from the more symmetric ST segment depression of ischemia; differentiation from ventricular hypertrophy with strain can sometimes be more problematic, especially since digitalis is frequently used in patients with congestive heart failure who often have left ventricular strain.

The digitalis effect usually is most prominent in leads with tall R waves. *Remember:* The digitalis effect is normal and predictable and does not necessitate discontinuing the drug.

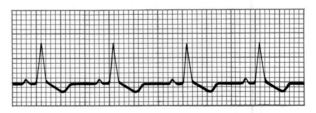

The digitalis effect, with asymmetric ST segment depression.

EKG Changes Associated With Toxic Blood Levels

The *toxic manifestations* of digitalis, on the other hand, may require clinical intervention. Digitalis intoxication can elicit conduction blocks and tachyarrhythmias, alone or in combination.

Conduction Blocks

Digitalis slows conduction through the AV node and can therefore cause first-, second-, and even third-degree AV block.

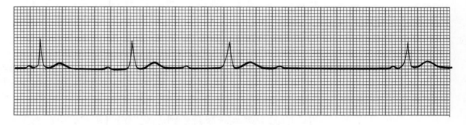

Wenckebach block caused by digitalis intoxication. The digitalis effect is not seen on this EKG.

The ability of digitalis to slow AV conduction has made it useful in the treatment of supraventricular tachycardias. For example, digitalis can slow the ventricular rate in patients with atrial fibrillation; in some patients, digitalis may even terminate the arrhythmia. Beta blockers, of which propranolol is the prototype, have a similar effect on AV conduction.

Tachyarrhythmias

There is no tachyarrhythmia that digitalis cannot cause. Paroxysmal atrial tachycardia (PAT) and PVCs are the most common; atrial flutter and fibrillation are the least common.

Combinations

The combination of PAT with second-degree AV block is the most characteristic rhythm disturbance of digitalis intoxication. The conduction block is usually 2:1, but may vary unpredictably. Digitalis is the most common, but not the only, cause of PAT with block.

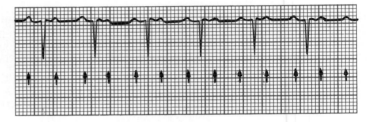

Paroxysmal atrial tachycardia (PAT) with 2 : 1 block. The arrows point to each P wave.

Quinidine

Quinidine, a commonly used antiarrhythmic drug, increases the QT interval and therefore can paradoxically increase the risk of ventricular tachyarrhythmias. The QT interval must be carefully monitored in all patients taking quinidine, and the drug should be stopped if substantial—usually more than 25%—prolongation occurs.

Other drugs that can increase the QT interval include other antiarrhythmic agents (*e.g.*, procainamide), the tricyclic antidepressants, and the phenothiazines.

In some patients taking quinidine, prominent U waves may develop. These do not require any adjustment in drug dosage.

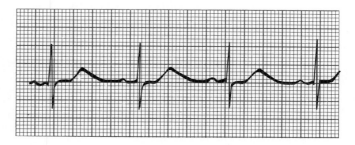

The prolonged QT interval on this tracing mandated reducing the quinidine dosage.

⊞ *Other Cardiac Disorders*

Pericarditis

Acute pericarditis may cause ST segment elevation and T wave flattening or inversion. These changes can easily be confused with an evolving infarction, as can the clinical picture. Certain features of the EKG can be helpful in differentiating pericarditis from infarction:

1. The ST segment and T wave changes in pericarditis tend to be diffuse (although not always), involving far more leads than the localized effect of infarction.

2. In pericarditis, T wave inversion usually occurs only after the ST segments have returned to baseline. In infarction, T wave inversion usually precedes normalization of the ST segments.

3. In pericarditis, Q wave formation does not occur.

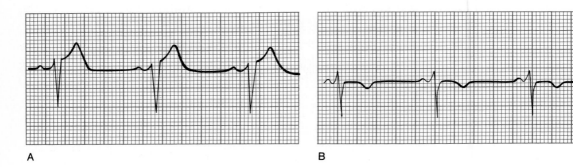

A   B

(*A*) Lead V$_3$ shows the ST segment elevation of acute pericarditis. (*B*) The same lead several days later shows that the ST segments have returned to baseline and the T waves have inverted. There are no Q waves.

Formation of a substantial *pericardial effusion* dampens the electrical output of the heart, resulting in low voltage in all leads. The ST segment and T wave changes of pericarditis may still be evident.

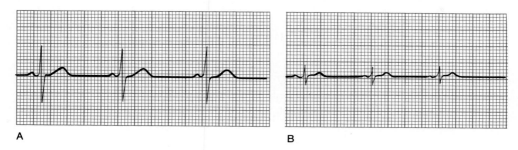

A   B

Lead I before (*A*) and after (*B*) the development of a pericardial effusion. Decreased voltage is the only significant change.

If an effusion is sufficiently large, the heart may actually rotate freely within the fluid-filled sac. This produces the phenomenon of *electrical alternans* in which the electrical axis of the heart varies with each beat. This can affect not only the axis of the QRS complex but that of the P and T waves as well. A varying axis is most easily recognized on the EKG by the varying amplitude of each waveform from beat to beat.

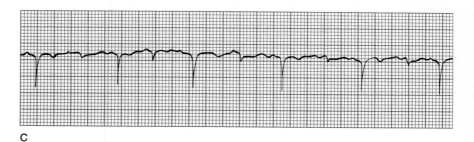

C

(*C*) Electrical alternans.

Hypertrophic Cardiomyopathy (Idiopathic Hypertrophic Subaortic Stenosis—IHSS)

We have already discussed IHSS in the case of Tom L. Many patients with IHSS have normal EKGs, but left ventricular hypertrophy and left axis deviation are not uncommon. Q waves may sometimes be seen laterally and occasionally inferiorly. These do not represent infarction.

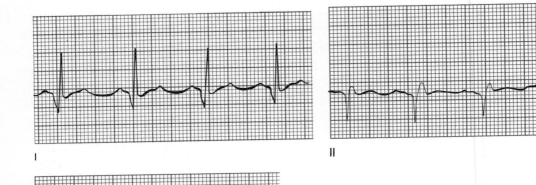

I

II

V5

IHSS. Significant Q waves can be seen in each of the three leads illustrated.

Myocarditis

Any diffuse inflammatory process involving the myocardium can produce a number of changes on the EKG. Most common are conduction blocks, especially bundle branch blocks and hemiblocks.

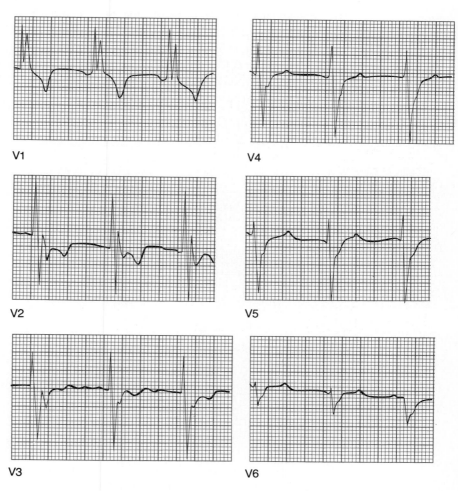

Right bundle branch block in a patient with active myocarditis following a viral infection.

⊞ *Pulmonary Disorders*

Chronic Obstructive Pulmonary Disease (COPD)

The EKG of a patient with long-standing emphysema may show low voltage, right axis deviation, and poor R wave progression in the precordial leads. The low voltage is caused by the dampening effects of the expanded residual volume of air trapped in the lungs. Right axis deviation is caused by the expanded lungs forcing the heart into a vertical or even rightward-oriented position.

COPD can lead to chronic cor pulmonale and right-sided congestive heart failure. The EKG may then show right atrial enlargement (P pulmonale) and right ventricular hypertrophy with strain.

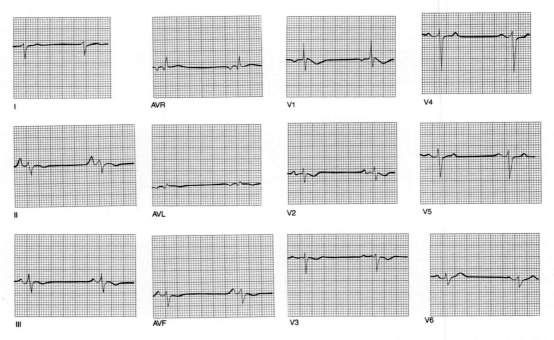

Chronic obstructive pulmonary disease. Note the low voltage, extreme right axis deviation, P pulmonale (in lead II), and precordial criteria for right ventricular hypertrophy.

Acute Pulmonary Embolism

A sudden massive pulmonary embolus can profoundly alter the EKG. Findings may include the following:

1. A pattern of right ventricular hypertrophy with strain, presumably due to acute right ventricular dilatation

2. Right bundle branch block

3. A large S wave in lead I and a deep Q wave in lead III. This is called the *S1Q3 pattern.* The T wave in lead III may also be inverted. Unlike an inferior infarction, in which Q waves are usually seen in at least two of the inferior leads, the Q waves in an acute pulmonary embolus are generally limited to lead III.

4. A number of arrhythmias may be produced. Most common are sinus tachycardia and atrial fibrillation.

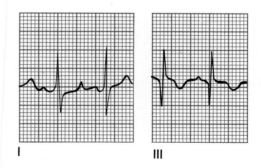

I   III

The S1Q3 pattern of a massive pulmonary embolus.

⊞ *Central Nervous System Disease*

Central nervous system (CNS) catastrophes, such as a subarachnoid bleed or cerebral infarction, can produce diffuse T wave inversion and prominent U waves. The T waves are typically very deep and very wide. Sinus bradycardia also is seen commonly. These changes are believed to be due to involvement of the autonomic nervous system.

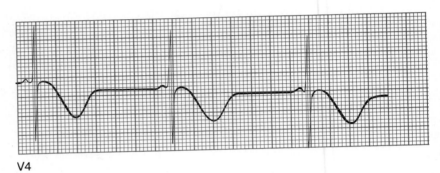

V4

Deeply inverted, wide T waves in lead V_4 in a patient with a central nervous system bleed.

⊞ *The Athlete's Heart*

Marathon runners and other athletes involved in endurance training that demands maximal aerobic capacity can develop alterations in their EKGs that can be quite unnerving if you are unfamiliar with them. These changes may include the following:

1. A resting sinus bradycardia, sometimes even below 30 beats per minute! Rather than a cause for concern, this profound sinus bradycardia is a testimony to the efficiency of their cardiovascular system.

2. Nonspecific ST segment and T wave changes. Typically, these consist of ST segment elevation in the precordial leads with T wave flattening or inversion.

3. Criteria for left ventricular hypertrophy and sometimes right ventricular hypertrophy.

4. Incomplete right bundle branch block.

5. Various arrhythmias, including junctional rhythms and a wandering atrial pacemaker.

6. First-degree or Wenckebach AV block.

None of these conditions are cause for concern, nor do they require treatment. More than one endurance athlete, undergoing a routine EKG, has been admitted to the CCU because of unfamiliarity with these changes.

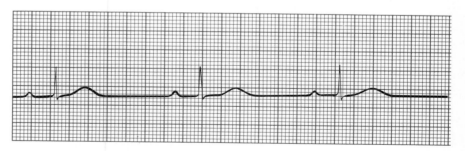

Sinus bradycardia and first-degree AV block in a triathlete.

Miscellaneous Conditions

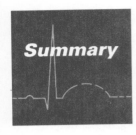
Summary

Electrolyte Disturbances

- *Hyperkalemia:* Evolution of (1) peaked T waves, (2) PR prolongation and P wave flattening, and (3) QRS widening. Ultimately, the QRS complexes and T waves merge to form a sine wave, and ventricular fibrillation may develop.

- *Hypokalemia:* ST depression, T wave flattening, U waves

- *Hypocalcemia:* Prolonged QT interval

- *Hypercalcemia:* Shortened QT interval

Hypothermia

- Osborne waves, prolonged intervals, sinus bradycardia, slow atrial fibrillation. Beware of muscle tremor artifact.

Drugs

- *Digitalis: Therapeutic levels* are associated with ST segment and T wave changes in leads with tall R waves; *toxic levels* are associated with tachyarrhythmias and conduction blocks; PAT with block is most characteristic.

- *Quinidine:* Prolonged QT interval, U waves

Other Cardiac Disorders

- *Pericarditis:* Diffuse ST segment and T wave changes. A large effusion can cause low voltage and electrical alternans.

- *IHSS:* Ventricular hypertrophy, left axis deviation, septal Q waves

- *Myocarditis:* Conduction blocks

Pulmonary Disorders

- *COPD:* Low voltage, right axis deviation, poor R wave progression. Chronic cor pulmonale can produce P pulmonale and right ventricular hypertrophy with strain.

- *Acute pulmonary embolism:* Right ventricular hypertrophy with strain, right bundle branch block, S1Q3. Sinus tachycardia and atrial fibrillation are the most common arrhythmias.

CNS Disease

- Diffuse T wave inversion, with T waves typically wide and deep; U waves

The Athlete's Heart

- Sinus bradycardia, nonspecific ST segment and T wave changes, left and right ventricular hypertrophy, incomplete right bundle branch block, first-degree or Wenckebach AV block, occasional supraventricular arrhythmia

Case 8

Amos T., a 25-year-old graduate student, is brought by ambulance to the emergency room, clutching his chest and looking not at all well. Vital signs show a blood pressure of 90/40 and an irregular pulse. His rhythm strip looks like this. Do you recognize the arrhythmia?

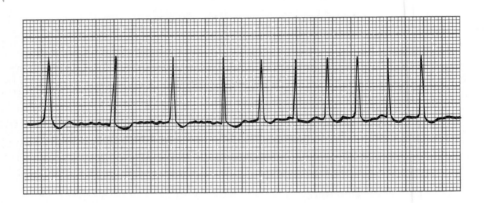

The patient is in atrial fibrillation.

Appropriate measures are taken and he is converted back to sinus rhythm, although his rate remains fast at 130 beats per minute. His blood pressure rises to 130/60. Despite successful conversion of his rhythm, he still complains of severe chest pain and shortness of breath. The emergency room physician wants to treat him immediately for an acute myocardial infarction, but you insist on a good 12-lead EKG first, a not unreasonable request since his vital signs are fairly stable. The EKG is obtained. Do you now agree with the emergency room physician's assessment?

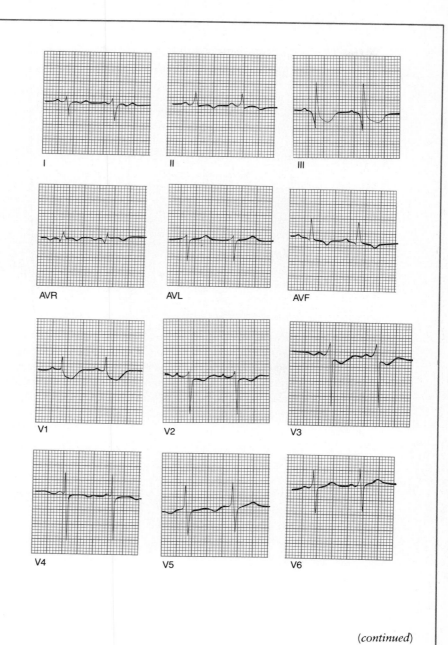

I II III

AVR AVL AVF

V1 V2 V3

V4 V5 V6

(continued)

Of course you don't. Hopefully, you noticed some of the following features:

1. The patient now has a rate of 100 beats per minute.

2. A pattern of right ventricular hypertrophy with strain is present.

3. A deep Q wave is seen in lead III and a deep S wave in lead II, the classic S1Q3 of an acute pulmonary embolus.

Do you now start jumping up and down and scream that the patient has an acute pulmonary embolus? No. You start jumping up and down and scream that the patient *may* have a pulmonary embolus. These EKG findings are suggestive but hardly conclusive. You have done your job well just by raising the issue; appropriate *diagnostic steps* can now be taken.

Amos is placed on intravenous heparin while awaiting his ventilation/perfusion scan. This is done within the hour and the diagnosis of a pulmonary embolism is confirmed. Amos remains in the hospital for 6 days of heparin therapy and is discharged home on oral anticoagulant therapy. There is no recurrence of his pulmonary embolism.

By the way, in case you were wondering why Amos developed a pulmonary embolism, you should know that he had a very strong family history of deep venous thrombophlebitis, and a careful hematologic work-up found that Amos had an inherited deficiency of protein S, a normal inhibitor of the coagulation cascade. Now, try to find *that* in other EKG books!

The Only EKG Book You'll Ever Need, second edition, by Malcolm S. Thaler. JB Lippincott Company, Philadelphia © 1995.

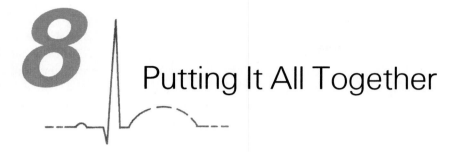

Putting It All Together

In this chapter you will learn:

1 a simple method to incorporate everything you have learned into a step-by-step analysis of any EKG

2 that all good things must come to an end, and we bid you a fond and overdue farewell!

And that is really all there is to it.

Well, perhaps not quite all. What we need now is a way to organize all of this information, a simple methodical approach that can be applied to each and every EKG. It is important that every EKG be approached in an orderly fashion, particularly while you are still new at this, so that nothing important is missed. As you read more and more cardiograms, what initially may seem forced and mechanical will pay big dividends and will soon seem like second nature.

Two admonitions:

1. *Know your patient.* It is true that EKGs can be read with fair accuracy in a little back room in total isolation, but the power of this tool only really emerges when it is integrated into a total clinical assessment.

2. *Read EKGs.* Then read some more. Read them wherever you can find them—in books, in papers, in patients' charts, on bathroom walls. And read other books; this may be the only EKG book you will ever need, but it should not be the only one you will ever *want* to read. There are many outstanding textbooks, each with something special to offer.

There are as many approaches to reading EKGs as there are cardiologists. Everyone ultimately arrives at a method that works best for him or her. The following 11-Step Method is probably no better and no worse than most others. The first four steps are largely data gathering. The remainder are directed at specific diagnoses.

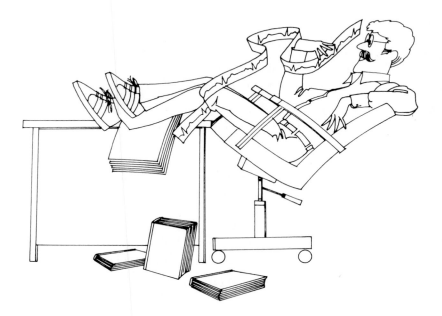

⊞ *The 11-Step Method for Reading EKGs*

Data Gathering

1. *Standardization.* Make sure the standardization mark on the EKG paper is 10 mm high so that 10 mm = 1 mV. Also make sure that the paper speed is correct.

2. *Heart rate.* Determine the heart rate by the quick three-step method described in Chapter 3.

3. *Intervals.* Measure the length of the PR and QT intervals and the width of the QRS complexes.

4. *QRS axis.* Is the axis normal, or is there axis deviation?

Diagnoses

5. *Rhythm.* Always ask The Four Questions:
    Are there P waves present?
    Are the QRS complexes wide or narrow?
    What is the relationship between the P waves and QRS complexes?
    Is the rhythm regular or irregular?

6. *AV block.* Apply the criteria in Chapter 4.

7. *Bundle branch block or hemiblock.* Apply the criteria in Chapter 4.

8. *Preexcitation.* Apply the criteria in Chapter 5.

(Note that steps 6 through 8 all involve looking for disturbances of conduction.)

9. *Enlargement and hypertrophy.* Apply the criteria for both atrial enlargement and ventricular hypertrophy.

10. *Coronary artery disease.* Look for Q waves and ST segment and T wave changes. Remember that not all such changes reflect coronary artery disease; know your differential diagnoses.

11. *Utter confusion.* Is there anything on the EKG you don't understand? Never hesitate to ask for assistance.

The following pages are "memory joggers." Cut them out and stick them in that little black book of medical pearls that you no doubt carry around with you. Cut them out anyway, even if you don't carry a little black book around with you; the exercise will do you good after sitting and staring bleary-eyed at this book for so long.

And if you are still thinking, "Is this really all there is to it?", the answer—reminding you that information only becomes knowledge with wisdom and experience—is, "Yes!"

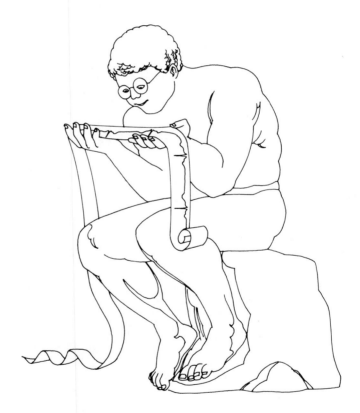

⊞ *Review Charts*

The 12 Leads

Anterior leads: V_1, V_2, V_3, V_4

Inferior leads: II, III, AVF

Left lateral leads: I, AVL, V_5, V_6,

AVR

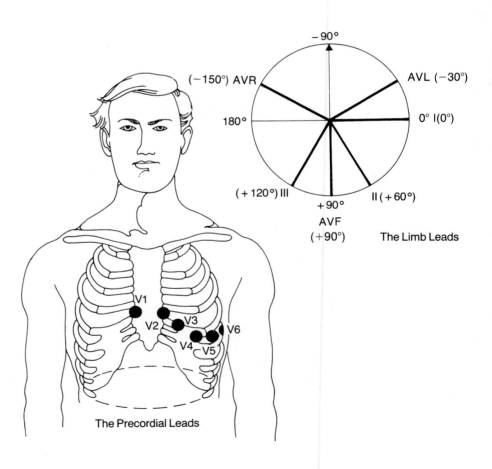

The Limb Leads

The Precordial Leads

Waves and Segments

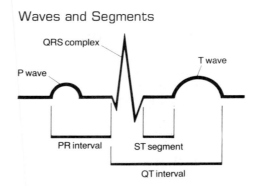

The heart is composed of pacemaker cells, electrical conducting cells, and myocardial cells. *Pacemaker cells* depolarize spontaneously and initiate each wave of depolarization. The SA node is usually the dominant pacemaker. *Electrical conducting cells* carry current rapidly and efficiently to distant regions of the heart. *Myocardial cells* constitute the bulk of the heart. When a wave of depolarization reaches a myocardial cell, calcium is released within the cell (excitation–contraction coupling), causing it to contract.

The *P wave* represents atrial depolarization. It is small and usually positive in the left lateral and inferior leads. It is often biphasic in leads III and V_1. Typically, it is most positive in lead II and most negative in lead AVR.

The *QRS complex* represents ventricular depolarization. It is usually predominantly positive in most lateral and inferior leads. Across the precordium, the R waves increase in size, progressing from V_1 to V_5. A small initial Q wave, representing septal depolarization, can often be seen in the left lateral and inferior leads.

The *T wave* represents ventricular repolarization. It is the most variable waveform, but it is usually positive in leads with tall R waves.

The *PR interval* represents the time from the start of atrial depolarization to the start of ventricular depolarization.

The *ST segment* represents the time from the end of ventricular depolarization to the start of ventricular repolarization.

The *QT interval* represents the time from the start of ventricular depolarization to the end of ventricular repolarization.

Calculating the Axis

	Lead I	*Lead AVF*
Normal axis	+	+
Left axis deviation	+	−
Right axis deviation	−	+
Extreme right axis deviation	−	−

Atrial Enlargement

Look at the P wave in leads II and V_1.

  Right atrial enlargement is characterized by the following:

1. Increased amplitude of the first portion of the P wave

2. No change in the duration of the P wave

3. Possible right axis deviation of the P wave.

  Left atrial enlargement is characterized by the following:

1. Occasionally, increased amplitude of the terminal component of the P wave

2. More consistently, increased P wave duration

3. No significant axis deviation.

Ventricular Hypertrophy

Look at the QRS complexes in all leads.

Right ventricular hypertrophy is characterized by the following:

1. Right axis deviation of greater than 100°

2. Ratio of R wave amplitude to S wave amplitude greater than 1 in V_1 and less than 1 in V_6.

Left ventricular hypertrophy is characterized by many criteria. The more that are present, the greater the likelihood that left ventricular hypertrophy is present. Precordial criteria include the following:

1. The R wave amplitude in V_5 or V_6 *plus* the S wave amplitude in V_1 or V_2 exceeds 35 mm.

2. The R wave amplitude in V_5 exceeds 26 mm.

3. The R wave amplitude in V_6 exceeds 18 mm.

4. The R wave amplitude in V_6 exceeds the R wave amplitude in V_5.

Limb lead criteria include the following:

1. The R wave amplitude in AVL exceeds 13 mm.

2. The R wave amplitude in AVF exceeds 21 mm.

3. The R wave amplitude in I exceeds 14 mm.

4. The R wave amplitude in I *plus* the S wave amplitude in III exceeds 25 mm.

The presence of strain (asymmetric ST segment depression and T wave inversion) indicates clinically significant hypertrophy, is most often seen in those leads with tall R waves, and may herald ventricular dilatation and failure.

The four basic types of arrhythmias are

1. Arrhythmias of sinus origin

2. Ectopic rhythms

3. Conduction blocks

4. Preexcitation syndromes.

Whenever you are interpreting the heart's rhythm, ask "The Four Questions":

1. Are P waves present?

2. Are the QRS complexes narrow (less than 0.12 seconds in duration) or wide (greater than 0.12 seconds)?

3. What is the relationship between the P waves and the QRS complexes?

4. Is the rhythm regular or irregular?

The answers for normal sinus rhythm are

1. Yes, P waves are present.

2. The QRS complexes are narrow.

3. There is one P wave for every QRS complex.

4. The rhythm is regular.

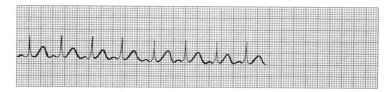

(A) Normal sinus rhythm.

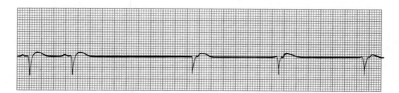

(B) Sinus tachycardia.

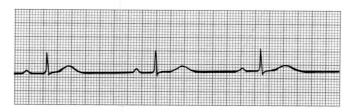

(C) Sinus bradycardia.

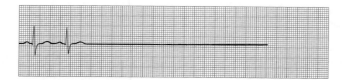

(D) Sinus arrest or exit block.

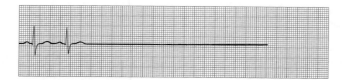

(E) Sinus arrest or exit block with junctional escape.

Supraventricular Arrhythmias

	Characteristics	*EKG*
PSVT	Regular Rate: 150 bpm–250 bpm Carotid massage: slows or terminates	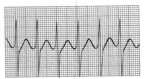

Flutter	Regular, sawtooth 2 : 1, 3 : 1, 4 : 1, etc., block Atrial rate: 250 bpm–350 bpm Ventricular rate: one half, one third, one fourth, etc., the atrial rate Carotid massage: increases block

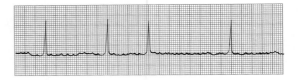

Fibrillation	Irregular Undulating baseline Atrial rate: 350 bpm–500 bpm Ventricular rate: variable Carotid massage: may slow ventricular rate

MAT	Irregular Rate: 100 bpm–200 bpm; sometimes less than 100 bpm Carotid massage: no effect

PAT	Regular Rate: 100 bpm–200 bpm Characteristic warm-up period in the automatic form Carotid massage: no effect, or only mild slowing

Ventricular Arrhythmias

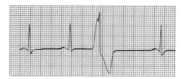

(A) PVCs.

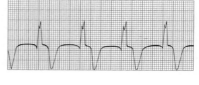

(D) Accelerated idioventricular rhythm.

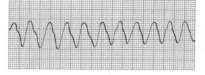

(B) Ventricular tachycardia.

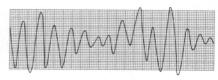

(E) Torsades de pointes.

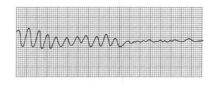

(C) Ventricular fibrillation.

Rules of Aberrancy

	VT	*PSVT*
Clinical Clues		
Carotid massage	No response	May terminate
Cannon a waves	May be present	Not seen
EKG Clues		
AV dissociation	May be seen	Not seen
Regularity	Slightly irregular	Very regular
Fusion beats	May be seen	Not seen
Initial QRS deflection	May differ from normal QRS complex	Same as normal QRS complex

A V Blocks

AV block is diagnosed by examining the relationship of the P waves to the QRS complexes.

1. *First degree:* The PR interval is greater than 0.2 seconds; *all* beats are conducted through to the ventricles.

2. *Second degree:* Only *some* beats are conducted through to the ventricles.

   a. *Mobitz type I (Wenckebach):* Progressive prolongation of the PR interval until a QRS is dropped

   b. *Mobitz type II:* All-or-nothing conduction, in which QRS complexes are dropped without PR interval prolongation

3. *Third degree:* No beats are conducted through to the ventricles. There is complete heart block with AV dissociation, in which the atria and ventricles are driven by independent pacemakers.

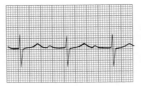
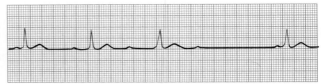

(*A*) First-degree AV block.   (*B*) Mobitz type I second-degree AV block (Wenckebach block).

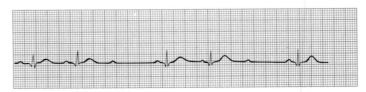

(*C*) Mobitz type II second-degree AV block.

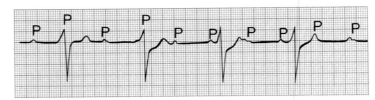

(*D*) Third-degree AV block.

Bundle Branch Blocks

Bundle branch block is diagnosed by looking at the width and configuration of the QRS complexes.

Criteria for Right Bundle Branch Block

1. QRS complex widened to greater than 0.12 seconds

2. RSR′ in leads V_1 and V_2 (rabbit ears) with ST segment depression and T wave inversion

3. Reciprocal changes in leads V_5, V_6, I, and AVL.

Criteria for Left Bundle Branch Block

1. QRS complex widened to greater than 0.12 seconds

2. Broad or notched R wave with prolonged upstroke in leads V_5, V_6, I, and AVL with ST segment depression and T wave inversion

3. Reciprocal changes in V_1 and V_2

4. Left axis deviation may be present.

Hemiblocks

Hemiblock is diagnosed by looking for left or right axis deviation.

Left Anterior Hemiblock

1. Normal QRS duration and no ST segment or T wave changes

2. Left axis deviation

3. No other cause of left axis deviation is present.

Left Posterior Hemiblock

1. Normal QRS duration and no ST segment or T wave changes

2. Right axis deviation

3. No other cause of right axis deviation is present.

Bifascicular Block

The features of right bundle branch block combined with left anterior hemiblock are as follows:

Right Bundle Branch Block

- QRS wider than 0.12 seconds
- RSR' in V_1 and V_2.

Left Anterior Hemiblock

- Left axis deviation.

The features of right bundle branch block combined with left posterior hemiblock are as follows:

Right Bundle Branch Block

- QRS wider than 0.12 seconds
- RSR' in V_1 and V_2.

Left Posterior Hemiblock

- Right axis deviation.

Preexcitation

Criteria for WPW Syndrome

1. PR interval less than 0.12 seconds

2. Wide QRS complexes

3. Delta wave seen in some leads.

Criteria for LGL Syndrome

1. PR interval less than 0.12 seconds

2. Normal QRS width

3. No delta wave.

   Arrhythmias commonly seen include the following:

1. Paroxysmal supraventricular tachycardia—narrow QRS complexes are more common than wide ones.

2. Atrial fibrillation—can be very rapid and can lead to ventricular fibrillation.

Myocardial Infarction

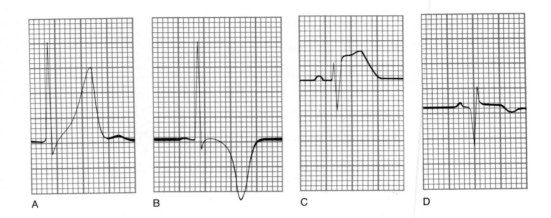

A   B   C   D

The diagnosis of a myocardial infarction is made by history, physical examination, serial cardiac enzyme determinations, and serial EKGs. During an acute infarction, the EKG evolves through three stages:

1. The T wave peaks (**A**), then inverts (**B**).

2. The ST segment elevates (**C**).

3. Q waves appear (**D**).

Criteria for Significant Q Waves

1. The Q wave must be greater than 0.04 seconds in duration.

2. The depth of the Q wave must be at least one third the height of the R wave in the same QRS complex.

Criteria for Non—Q Wave Infarctions

1. T wave inversion.

2. ST segment depression persisting for more than 48 hours in the appropriate setting.

Localizing the Infarct

Inferior infarction: leads II, III, and AVF

Often caused by occlusion of the right coronary artery or its descending branch

Reciprocal changes in anterior and left lateral leads.

Lateral infarction: leads I, AVL, V_5, and V_6

Often caused by occlusion of the left circumflex artery
Reciprocal changes in inferior leads.

Anterior infarction: any of the precordial leads (V_1 through V_6)

Often caused by occlusion of the left anterior descending artery
Reciprocal changes in inferior leads.

Posterior infarction: reciprocal changes in lead V_1 (ST-segment depression, tall R wave)

Often caused by occlusion of the right coronary artery.

The ST Segment

ST segment *elevation* may be seen

1. With an evolving infarction

2. In Prinzmetal's angina.

ST segment *depression* may be seen

1. With typical exertional angina

2. In a non-Q wave infarction.

ST depression is also one indicator of a positive stress test.

Miscellaneous EKG Changes

Electrolyte Disturbances

- *Hyperkalemia:* Evolution of peaked T waves, PR prolongation and P wave flattening, and QRS widening. Ultimately, the QRS complexes and T waves merge to form a sine wave, and ventricular fibrillation may develop.

- *Hypokalemia:* ST depression, T wave flattening, U waves

- *Hypocalcemia:* Prolonged QT interval

- *Hypercalcemia:* Shortened QT interval

Hypothermia

- Osborne waves, prolonged intervals, sinus bradycardia, slow atrial fibrillation; beware of muscle tremor artifact.

Drugs

- *Digitalis:* Therapeutic levels associated with ST segment and T wave changes in leads with tall R waves; toxic levels associated with tachyarrhythmias and conduction blocks; PAT with block is most characteristic.

- *Quinidine:* Prolonged QT interval, U waves

Other Cardiac Disorders

- *Pericarditis:* Diffuse ST segment and T wave changes. A large effusion can cause low voltage and electrical alternans.

- *IHSS:* Ventricular hypertrophy, left axis deviation, septal Q waves

- *Myocarditis:* Conduction blocks

Pulmonary Disorders

- *COPD:* Low voltage, right axis deviation, poor R wave progression. Chronic cor pulmonale can produce P pulmonale and right ventricular hypertrophy with strain.

- *Acute pulmonary embolism:* Right ventricular hypertrophy with strain, right bundle branch block, S1Q3. Sinus tachycardia and atrial fibrillation are the most common arrhythmias.

CNS Disease

- Diffuse T wave inversion, with T waves typically wide and deep; U waves

The Athlete's Heart

- Sinus bradycardia, nonspecific ST segment and T wave changes, left and right ventricular hypertrophy, incomplete right bundle branch block, first-degree or Wenckebach AV block, occasional supraventricular arrhythmia

Index

Page numbers followed by f *indicate figures; those followed by* t *indicate tabular material.*